Piecing the Puzzle

Piecing the Puzzle

THE GENESIS OF AIDS RESEARCH IN AFRICA

LARRY KROTZ

UNIVERSITY OF MANITOBA PRESS

University of Manitoba Press
Winnipeg, Manitoba
Canada R3T 2M5
uofmpress.ca

Printed in Canada
Text printed on chlorine-free, 100% post-consumer recycled paper

16 15 14 13 12   1 2 3 4 5

Cover design: David Drummond
Cover photo by Cheryl Albuquerque
Interior design: Jessica Koroscil

Library and Archives Canada Cataloguing in Publication

Krotz, Larry, 1948–
Piecing the puzzle : the genesis of
AIDS research in Africa / Larry Krotz.

Includes bibliographical references and index.
ISBN 978-0-88755-730-9 (pbk.)
ISBN 978-0-88755-420-9 (PDF e-book)
ISBN 978-0-88755-422-3 (epub e-book)

1. AIDS (Disease) — Research — Kenya. 2. AIDS
(Disease) — International cooperation. I. Title.

RA643.86.K4K76 2012   362.196'97920096762   C2011-908245-4

The University of Manitoba Press gratefully acknowledges the financial
support for its publication program provided by the Government of Canada
through the Canada Book Fund, the Canada Council for the Arts, the Manitoba
Department of Culture, Heritage, Tourism, the Manitoba Arts Council,
and the Manitoba Book Publishing Tax Credit.

FSC
www.fsc.org
MIX
Paper from
responsible sources
FSC® C016245

Contents

Photographs follow pages 80 and 126

Acknowledgements

This book would never have come to fruition without a great deal of help from many quarters. First on that list is Allan Ronald. Allan is, of course, a central character in the story, it being his connections in 1980 with Nairobi's Herbert Nsanze that started the scientific collaboration which became the tale the book tells. But the book itself would not have happened without Allan's energy and generosity. From the moment I approached him with the idea of setting down the history of what I have always thought was an extraordinary episode in not just Canadian but global scientific research—and around the most explosive epidemic of our times—he was enthusiastic. He provided all his information, introduced me to other vital sources and, most important, shook the money trees for the support I needed for research and writing. Allan, Frank Plummer, and Stephen Moses not only met with me many times to explain their work and how the story, as they saw it, had unfolded, but they also double-checked my material to ascertain that what I had was accurate, not only historically but also medically and scientifically. Many others gave selflessly of information and perspective, notably Joanne Embree and Ian Maclean. At the administrative end, Carol Sigurdson and Stacey Zazula were on top of making sure my expenses got covered.

It has been a pleasure to work once again with the University of Manitoba Press. The support of David Carr, the encouragement of Cheryl Miki, and the trusted editorial hand of Glenn Bergen have been invaluable. As have been the comments during the writing process of my at-hand readers, Jim Rothwell and my ever-patient wife Stephanie Leontowitsch.

The photographs in the book come predominantly from the cameras of Cheryl Albuquerque and Rupert Kaul, both of whom bring incredible insights to the canvas of Nairobi and its HIV clinics.

Note on Sources

T he introduction will explain that this is a story I've been following as a journalist, author, and documentary filmmaker since 1992. As you can imagine, I have many years' worth of notes. The book is based partly on notes taken over those years, but specifically and very substantially on information gleaned from interviews conducted in 2009, 2010, and 2011 with a great number of individuals who are central to the story. Among these are three researchers in particular who have been deeply involved in the collaboration between the University of Manitoba and Nairobi since, in one case, the very beginning in 1980, and in the other two instances from very near the beginning. I met with Allan Ronald, Frank Plummer, and Stephen Moses literally dozens of times in Winnipeg, Toronto, and Nairobi, at Stephen's cottage on Lake of the Woods, as well as exchanging numerous e-mails. On top of that, on four visits to Winnipeg I interviewed Joanne Embree, Leslie Slaney, Ian Maclean, Theresa Birkholz, Neil Simonsen, Margaret Fast, Keith Fowke, Blake Ball, and Arnold Naimark. In Toronto I interviewed Kelly MacDonald and Rupert Kaul. In January 2010 I travelled to Nairobi, Kenya, where I interviewed King Holmes, Marleen Temmerman, Robert Bailey, Larry Gelmon, Joshua Kimani, Omu Anzala, Elizabeth Ngugi, Ann Maingi, Jane Kamene, J.O. Ndinya-Achola, Walter Joako, Loe Dierick, and Benson Estambale. In the spring of 2010 I went to London to interview Peter Piot and Oxford to interview Sarah Rowland-Jones. I carried out e-mail interviews with Joan Kreiss in California, Grace John-Stewart in Seattle, Herbert Nsanze in Uganda, and Carla Plummer in Winnipeg. Gary Slutkin, David Haase, Robert Brunham, and Myrna Ronald were interviewed by telephone.

In the summer of 2008 I attended the World AIDS Conference in Mexico City. Some material comes from presentations and panel discussions at that event.

Piecing the Puzzle

Introduction

Diseases, especially those that kill us, are something we humans obsess about keenly. To do so is a natural part of trying to survive. We are conscious of the fact that death somehow, some day awaits us, and wonder persistently if we can do anything about that. What can take us down, either individually or as a group? Who is in charge of fighting it off? We have, in this vein, spent the last half century preoccupied with cancer and heart disease, killers in the aging West; malaria and cholera, scourges in the tropics; multiple sclerosis, a debilitating disease hitting the all-too-young; Alzheimer's, infecting the burgeoning demographic of the old. But an entirely different kind of disease is the one that can both kill us and be spread from person to person in the form of a contagious epidemic. The example that in our lifetime stands out above anything else is AIDS. Since first appearing in the early 1980s, Acquired Immune Deficiency Syndrome has encompassed everything about both disease and epidemic that humans find profoundly unsettling. Its arc over three decades has been perplexing and fearsome. It was mysterious, coming on the scene in one part of the world—first diagnosed in North American cities among gay men and then intravenous drug users—and then showing up in massive numbers in another part of the world, sub-Saharan Africa, to affect a completely different population, male and female heterosexuals, as well as the babies of infected women.

AIDS was always considered fearsome, in part because it was a new and unknown quantity, something that could pop up anywhere to kill its victims without mercy. But AIDS was fearsome as well because it was understood immediately as a disease that was transmitted sexually (though it is spread likewise through blood in transfusions as well as by shared needles). Sexual transmission is what settled in the lurid imagination and, like sexually transmitted diseases before it, AIDS spawned prejudice and engendered a particular kind of shame. This both doubly burdened its victims and truncated an effective public response; people hid their symptoms from friends, families, and health care professionals, and the nasty terrain of stigmatization inhibited the effectiveness of public health efforts. In the early days, rampant speculation and the resulting fear was almost out of control. In early 1987, the U.S. Secretary of Health and Human Services predicted that the worldwide HIV/AIDS epidemic would eventually make the Black Death, which wiped out between a third and a half of the population of Europe, seem "pale by comparison."[1]

HIV/AIDS was, and continues to be, recalcitrant and frustrating. It has persistently defied attempts to do what medical science and public health practitioners most like to do—find a way to contain a threat through preventative measures, inoculate against it with a vaccine, and ultimately find a cure. One of the problems is that AIDS is not a disease or an illness per se, but a medical condition whose consequences are a spectrum of illnesses, so-called opportunistic infections that invade when the body's immune system is weak and, in the end, kill the patient. The other problem is the clever mutability of the virus that has defied all attempts to place it in a single box. For the full life of the epidemic, a vaccine has been held out as the silver bullet against its continued spread. This vaccine continues to be elusive, as is a cure, though the entire context for fighting the disease did change dramatically in the late 1990s, especially in the well-off West, with the discovery of combination antiretroviral therapies. These helped patients escape the almost-certain death sentence that HIV infection had meant up until then and allowed them to continue to live their lives, knowing that HIV infection is survivable at least in the short—and it seems increasingly the middle—term. The therapies, however, are expensive and challenging to distribute, which means that though AIDS as a crisis was diminished in North America, the therapies did not have the same impact in the part of the world where the epidemic had by then become far more virulent, eastern and southern Africa.

AIDS, which was immediately designated a "crisis," was so exotic it might have come to us from outer space. The responses reflected that mindset. In the lavish labs of the National Institutes of Health (NIH) in Washington and at UCLA, in infinitely more modest labs and clinics in Kampala and Johannesburg and Nairobi, medical scientists struggled to come to terms with the mystery and tame its ferocity. In many ways they invented the response, having at hand technologies—like airplane travel and computers—that had not been available for previous epidemics. Doctors and researchers and policy makers who worked for international organizations packed their bags and bought plane tickets and set up shop far away from home. Universities that believed they had special skill sets—or individual researchers who were highly motivated—set out to put those skills to work and form partnerships with others. The responses were imperfect to be sure, never speedy enough in the opinions of some, too haphazard in the view of others. Either too expensive or, since money was always an issue, not lavish enough. And the fact that the threat of HIV/AIDS still continues means that there was not the level of success that might have been wished. But those in pursuit set forth with inventiveness, persistence, diligence, and humanity. Frustrations followed breakthroughs that in turn followed frustrations, and in this manner research lurched along. In the end, though thirty years on HIV/AIDS has yet to be "conquered," all the work has produced at least two achievements. One is an infinitely deeper understanding of the disease itself, its epidemiology, as well as the human immune system it attacks. The other equally important development is a growing understanding of how researchers and caregivers can best work together—across international boundaries, across cultures, and across time zones. The new field of "global health" and the practice of "global health collaborations" came into being as HIV/AIDS researchers learned how to turn potential rivals into colleagues and how to secure labs and grants and cohorts in places far from home. This book, by telling the story of one front in the battle against HIV/AIDS, will try to explore both of these phenomena. What I want to do is to place one single initiative—what I describe as the "Nairobi collaboration"—into the context of the larger HIV/AIDS epidemic, and to look at the historic epidemic through the eyes of this discrete initiative, that both encompassed and had to face up to what others everywhere were encountering.

In January 2008, when *Time* magazine published its annual list of everything important, number one among world-shaking scientific discoveries of the previous year was something achieved by a group of health researchers, including some from a university in the middle of the Canadian prairies. In a far corner of Kenya, Winnipeg's University of Manitoba—in a partnership that included the University of Nairobi and the University of Illinois—had run a clinical trial that determined that circumcised men were at least 60 percent less likely than uncircumcised men to acquire HIV during sex with women.

Over the previous five years a team led by Stephen Moses, a Toronto-born MD and public health researcher, and his colleagues Robert Bailey, an anthropologist from Chicago and J.O. Ndinya-Achola, a microbiologist from Nairobi, had studied 2,700 young Luo men who live on the shores of the fabled Lake Victoria. They and their Kenyan colleagues had circumcised half the young men and observed, for a period of two years, their HIV infection rates along with those who had not been circumcised. The numbers, when they started to come in, were so startling that the safety board that oversees such scientific trials insisted it didn't need any more information. The trial was stopped before completion, circumcision was offered to everybody, and the procedure was added to the worldwide standard of HIV/AIDS preventative care.[2]

Instantly, circumcision moved from the fringes of the formerly skeptical AIDS-research world to the very centre. Bill Clinton singled it out in his speech to the International AIDS Conference; Bill Gates turned on the money tap; and finally came anointment by *Time* magazine. Henceforth, along with vaccine research, condom use, and antiretroviral treatments, circumcision would take its place on the stage in the battle against the global pandemic of HIV/AIDS. "In areas where HIV-1 prevalence constitute a generalized population epidemic," stated an editorial in the prestigious British medical journal the *Lancet*, "male circumcision could have a dramatic life-saving effect."[3]

This was not the first time work by a small group of Canadian scientists based in Winnipeg had leapt to the attention of those following the dreadful story of HIV/AIDS. Back in the early 1990s, researching an article in a dusty corner of Zimbabwe, I requested clippings from a librarian in a little outpost office. I was flabbergasted when reference after reference cited statistics and figures credited to the University of Manitoba. The mid-sized Canadian school, back in my hometown, was second only to Baltimore's Johns Hopkins University as a world authority on AIDS. In Africa, the well-kept secret was that it was considered number one. Neither was it the first time this group of Canadian scientists had triumphed in ways that can best be described as working against prevailing conventional wisdom. During a period of almost thirty years, since the early 1980s, the group had built a careful relationship with the East African country of Kenya around research and clinical support. The cumulative enterprise, involving hundreds of Canadians, Americans, Europeans, and Kenyans, produced some extraordinary discoveries that filled critical gaps in the puzzle that is HIV/AIDS. Their research was central to explaining circumcision's vital role in preventing HIV/AIDS. But they had also told the world how HIV was transmitted to the newborn babies of infected mothers—sometimes through breast milk; how using oral contraception made some women more rather than less susceptible to HIV; and how HIV took advantage of opportunities offered by other sexually transmitted diseases to make its entry into the body. Finally, they had come upon the most unlikely of phenomena, a group of workers in the sex trade who did not become infected with HIV, which caused the scientists to turn their thoughts and research to what the immunity of a group of special women might mean for everyone.

This is a story I became acquainted with personally in 1993, when I first met the various participants in Nairobi. As a journalist and filmmaker I then quite persistently followed them and their work right through to 2010. In those seventeen years I paid numerous visits to Nairobi, Mombasa, and Kisumu and felt both overawed and privileged to have such ready access to both an extraordinary venture of medical science and one of the defining catastrophes of history.[4] I was able to witness the AIDS epidemic through very localized eyes, making my perspective, admittedly, somewhat one-dimensional. But the front-row seat, if you will, compensated by allowing the macro to be seen through the lens of the micro. All the local frustrations and struggles I considered invaluable to our being able to understand the story of the bigger battle were played out by the characters right in front of me. One important detail I noted through it all was how all the achievements were made not by individuals acting on their own, but through delicately engineered collaborations, partnerships that stretched across worlds, traditions, and even generations. Purveyors of Western medical science, despite its exalted status, were obliged to engage in a careful dance with local mores and customs. Collaborations between individuals from a variety of countries and institutions, including the host, Kenya, had to be developed, and everybody had to learn to work together. Their accomplishment was also a demonstration of science and the scientist at work, facing challenges, enduring pressures and frustrations, enjoying periodic triumphs. And every morning, returning to the task.

"Science," writes Elizabeth Pisani in her book, *The Wisdom of Whores: Bureaucrats, Brothels, and the Business of AIDS,* "does not exist in a vacuum. It exists in a world of money and votes, a world of media enquiry and lobbyists, of pharmaceutical manufacturing and environmental activism and religions and political ideologies and all the other complexities of human life."[5] This is one aspect of science, and an important one. But science is also haphazard, serendipitous, and a matter of being in the right place at the right time to ask the right—sometimes counterintuitive—questions. Timing, perseverance, luck, perspicacity, and that most nuanced of commodities, opportunity, are also vital. Often, a scientist doing research starts down a road having no idea where it will ultimately lead, but proceeds anyway, propelled by faith in his or her own curiosity and the hunger to contribute to both the fund of knowledge and the well-being of the world. These are lofty aims, and they are the ones that make this a story worth telling.

The history of science is likewise the story of some important "ifs": if Archimedes had not over-filled his bath, if Isaac Newton had not seated himself beneath the apple tree at that particular moment. Historians of AIDS might also speculate how things would be different had a doctor named Allan Ronald from that middle Canadian city of Winnipeg not run into a fellow medical researcher, Herbert Nsanze, at a propitious moment in 1980. Ronald, well-known among infectious diseases specialists for having unlocked the secrets of an ugly genital ulcer disease known as chancroid, was approached after a conference by his counterpart, Herbert Nsanze, head of the medical microbiology department at the University of Nairobi. "Come to Kenya," Nsanze pleaded, "and help us with our sexual diseases problem." Ronald, the kind of man who rarely turns down the chance to board an airplane, went to Kenya, parlaying that trip into a series of future visits and a formal relationship between his University of Manitoba and Nsanze's University of Nairobi. Money followed for the construction of labs and clinics and, most important, to support travel back and forth of students, some of whom would stay for years and become, like Frank Plummer, who eventually took charge of the project and lived in Kenya for seventeen years, eminently well-known names in the annals of global health research. You can call it luck or you can call it fate; either way, being in the right place at the right time put the Canadians at the epicentre of the AIDS epidemic right from its very beginning. But the intriguing part of the story is also how they stuck it out during the countless times when it would have been easier to pack up and leave. They fought for funding and continually negotiated their place in the East African community.

This book is the story of how unlikely things happen. It is also a look at how things might have been different. The HIV/AIDS epidemic that terrified the world and devastated great swaths of Africa is now solidly into its second generation. This has made it, at long last, the property not just of epidemiologists but of historians. These historians are beginning to look at the facts and the myths, the truisms and the conventional wisdoms, that kept everything and everyone going during the intense years of the fight. Given the luxury of hindsight, some of the trajectory is bound to be altered, questioned, or revised.[6]

At the International AIDS Conference in Mexico City in the summer of 2008, those involved in every aspect of the global plague (some 22,000 delegates) met for the seventeenth time. As they milled about the sprawling halls and corridors of Mexico City's Banamex Convention Centre, taking in the hundreds of displays and encountering old friends and colleagues, the delegates noted how the human rights of people suffering from HIV/AIDS were as high on the agenda as were science and pharmaceuticals. Panel after panel was going to discuss unfair impositions like international travel restrictions on people with HIV/AIDS. This was important because human rights had become a staple of the meetings, but it was counterbalanced by something novel at this congress: increasingly frank discussions about the failures of the last twenty-five years. Richard Horton, editor of the *Lancet,* chaired a panel that called for something not much heard at recent AIDS conferences: "action to form and sustain," as the agenda put it, "a new prevention movement that will push prevention efforts beyond the current levels." "It is widely acknowledged," Horton grimly admitted to the ensuing panel, "that we cannot treat our way out of the HIV pandemic." Stefano Bertozzi, head of HIV prevention for Mexico, was blunter still, charging that "billions of dollars were spent on what should have been an easily preventable disease."

Everybody who pays attention throughout the world knows the numbers: 40 million deaths and counting and 33.3 million people living with HIV, with sub-Saharan Africa still representing 68 percent of the infected (more than 22 million) and nearly three-quarters of all AIDS deaths.[7] The most recent report on the global HIV/AIDS epidemic issued by UNAIDS states that while the percentage of people living with HIV has stabilized since 2000, the overall numbers have increased as a result of new infections and the beneficial effects of more widely available antiretroviral therapy. People are not dying as quickly as in the past, but new people continue to get infected—including 2.6 million estimated new infections in 2009.[8]

The verdict of history will doubtless make clear where opportunities were missed as well as where there was tardiness in responding to the greatest infectious disease epidemic the world has known. History will also pronounce on the other great failure: that it took far too long to grapple with how devastating the plague could be for the world's poorest regions. What will we see when we look at the HIV/AIDS epidemic with the benefit of this 20-20 hindsight? There will be lessons, for sure; tales of heroism, no doubt; but also stories that will cause chagrin. The Canadians and all their African, American, British, and Belgian partners coordinated their research and published their findings—sometimes findings that took the world a bit of time to swallow. And they kept working. Nothing, as anybody who followed the AIDS crisis knows, happened quickly. Nor was AIDS an epidemic that welcomed prophets. Which leads to what historians of the epidemic are going to have to weigh: is it truly the case that if some of the voices from the front lines of the epidemic had been listened to things could have been different? Infectious disease epidemiology has developed over centuries as human populations time after time faced assaults from viral or bacterial infections. Each war—for battle is the metaphor most employed to describe the contests between humans and SARS or humans and tuberculosis or humans and smallpox—is a new one fought on its own terms. But over time principles of behaviour and strategy, from quarantine to vaccine, have been developed with the goals of containing and beating epidemics. How did those approaches play out with HIV/AIDS?

In some cases, probably not as well as they should have. "This disease could have been prevented, we knew how to do it," claims Frank Plummer, one of those who had a ringside seat through the first decades of the epidemic and now have the benefit of hindsight. His assessment is a stark one and probably not welcomed by those in charge of thirty years' worth of policy. But it is an important observation reflecting the frustrations experienced over and over by those trying to push strategies forward while up to their elbows in devastation.

Circumcision is a case in point. Most dismaying when one thinks about male circumcision as a strategy for HIV/AIDS prevention is the story of how long it took and of the stubborn hurdle-filled journey to get the procedure and its effects accepted by the big thinkers and the big agencies in the global AIDS effort. The first evidence of circumcision's efficacy became available in the 1980s, close to the outbreak of HIV/AIDS, in no small part unearthed by efforts of the University of Manitoba scientists and their colleagues working in Kenya. Their research tweaked their interest in a possible connection between circumcision and reduced transmission of the virus, which they shared in at least four articles in highly placed medical journals between 1988 and 1991.[9] The case they developed included repeated clinical observations that circumcised men had lower HIV prevalence, plus a correspondence of lower HIV infection rates in parts of African countries where circumcision was a traditional practice. The statistics they laid out should have been persuasive. This was seventeen years before the results of their clinical trials would be published in the *Lancet*, along with its editorial praising them and their work. What happened during those seventeen lost years is, as much as anything, a study in the ineptness with which the great HIV/AIDS epidemic has been handled by the world bodies in charge of controlling or eliminating it. As critics point out, "male circumcision offers more effective protection against HIV than any of the experimental vaccines currently undergoing clinical trials around the world. It is also cheaper, carries fewer side effects, requires no booster shots, and is available now."[10] Male circumcision also indirectly protects women because reducing HIV prevalence in men means women are less likely to be exposed to the virus. Yet it was not until 2000 that the first trials were organized, and comprehensive circumcision as a strategy is only now becoming widely adopted more than twenty years after the first arguments were made.

The value of the work done over the two and a half decades of the AIDS epidemic by the Nairobi collaboration is underscored by Stephen Moses's observation that "four or five key technologies into transmission and prevention of HIV/AIDS all originated from research in our Kenyan program." But the shortcomings of the battle against the pandemic also get aired via Frank Plummer's blunt assessment: "I would be one of those who say this epidemic could have, should have been prevented," he said in an interview for this book. "Why did it take twenty years to get to circumcision? I don't think you could have prevented it [the AIDS epidemic] totally, but it could have been a lot better. We knew by the late '80s the cornerstones of good prevention: get prostitutes to use condoms, treat STDs, circumcise men, don't have kids breast-feed for years and years. Some of [the world-level policy makers in charge of addressing the epidemic] got it, others did not."

CHAPTER ONE

Waging War With Infectious Diseases

J anuary at the Equator is the height of summer. In Nairobi, the capital of Kenya, the sun shines fiercely, though the days, if you find shade, are extraordinarily pleasant and the nights exquisite. Rains in December have greened everything up and now this city of 3 million, with its mix of old British style colonial buildings, middle-class estates, and crammed, tin-roofed shantytowns with open sewers only short distances from bucolic avenues lined with diplomats' estates, is busy and thriving. A striking presence is that of the Chinese. Throughout Africa, the world's newest superpower is busy extracting resources and donating physical projects. Here in Nairobi, through completely gutted sections of downtown, the Chinese government is building an eight-lane highway heading north. Near the airport you pass beneath an arch of friendship erected between the peoples of China and Kenya, a symbol of things present and enticingly—or ominously—to come. Otherwise the great mill of life goes on much as always, labourers lugging heavily loaded handcarts struggle through intersections next to smoke-belching lorries and shiny air-conditioned Land Rovers. At a nicely appointed hotel on the edge of downtown, another reality of Kenyan life is about to unfold: a scientific meeting on HIV/AIDS.

On Monday morning participants start to gather. Four hundred are expected over the course of five days. Today nurses and doctors who last week toiled inside the smudged walls of shantytown clinics with patients queued down the dark hallways, line up themselves—for tea and coffee by the swimming pool bar of the Mayfair Court. John Mungai, whom I last saw crammed sideways into his cubbyhole office at the Baba Dogo clinic on the far side of town where he counsels men about to get HIV tests, is hardly recognizable, smiling broadly in his spiffy suit. Laboratory technicians have disembarked from buses boarded long hours ago at the far ends of the country, from Kisumu, west on the shores of Lake Victoria, and Mombasa, by the Indian Ocean. Professors in the medical school at the University of Nairobi have told their students they'll be away for a couple of days.

Foreign visitors are here as well and will make up about a third of the assembly. It used to be almost all foreigners, and the fact that there are now so many (mostly young) Kenyan faces among the participants is a true testament to some of the event's signature achievements—inclusiveness and mentoring. But the foreigners come too—escaping winter in the northern hemisphere—guaranteeing the uniqueness and strength of the event, that it is most definitively a two-way enterprise. Researchers have arrived from Canada—Winnipeg, Vancouver, Ottawa, and Toronto; from the U.S.—Seattle, Chicago, San Francisco. And from Europe—the U.K., Belgium, and Sweden. Old hands who have been coming here every January since the late 1980s mingle with young scientists who were mere infants in those early days of the meeting. The Annual Review Meeting 2010 of the University of Nairobi STD/AIDS Collaborative Group will listen to 118 presentations, almost all of which will describe work in progress. Some, indeed, is research that will never see publication, but what is important is the opportunity to share the work, to get feedback from colleagues and senior scientists, some of them giants in the field. This is not properly a conference, but a meeting, though the old-timers still call it a "retreat," which is how it began twenty years ago when there weren't 400 participants but only a couple of dozen. "We insisted the big shots come together all at the same time so we could present our work to them and to each other," recalls Marleen Temmerman, who has come from Belgium. In the 1980s Temmerman—whose down-to-earth demeanour belies her lofty credentials as a top-tier researcher—was a youthful obstetrician newly arrived for a stint in Kenya that would stretch into eight years. Now her resume is gilded: head of the department of obstetrics at Ghent University Hospital, a nominee for the lifetime achievement award granted by the *British Medical Journal*, and, to boot, a senator in the Belgian Parliament. She maintains her hand in Kenya through her position as director of the International Centre for Reproductive Health (ICHR). Temmerman travels with two journalists from Brussels who are preparing a newspaper feature about her.

As things get underway, it becomes readily apparent that presenters are approaching the vast subject of HIV/AIDS from all sides. The research papers, each of which will be given a fifteen-minute treatment, are as diverse as "Risk factors and potential intervention targets in HIV-1 discordant couples," which struggles with the problem of limiting HIV spread when one partner is infected and the other is not, and "Male circumcision for HIV prevention in Nyanza," which marshals research to assess the success of the prevention strategy of circumcising young men. Doctors from Winnipeg who have spent more than a decade poring over the genetic profile of HIV-resistant sex workers in attempts to learn more about the mysteries of the immune system will deliver their thoughts: "Setting up multiple barricades along the HIV infection pathway." A contingent of anthropologists from the universities of Illinois and Nairobi who have been trying to figure out how to intervene around cultural practices that are risky for HIV spread will present: "Widow inheritance and sexual networks in Siaya District." Anthropology and sociology mix with biology and microbiology. A group of Kenyans and Canadians will describe their efforts to get people to use cell phones (ubiquitous here now, even among the poor) to stay in touch with clinics and manage their health, in particular, keeping them regular with regard to the daily ingestion of their antiretroviral therapies. The audiences are earnest and attentive, and empty chairs are hard to find in the darkened conference room during the long mornings and afternoons. Outside, on the patios of the hotel complex, the work goes on non-stop. Whatever the first meeting might have looked like two decades ago, it would not have been governed, as this one is, by the laptop. One of the most dramatic changes is technology; it is now somehow the most satisfying of all possible worlds to be in your room, in a coffee shop, or seated at a table by the pool, thousands of kilometres—in some cases ten time zones—away from home with your entire office available from inside the little machine in front of you. BlackBerrys are everywhere, with nary a pencil or sheet of paper to be seen. Projected on screens in every meeting room, charts, pie graphs, and numbers are the uniform currency of science, used at one end to prove a point and, at the other, to raise grant money.

The meeting itself is about one main thing, making progress in the war on a disease that has traumatized Kenya, as it has all of southern Africa. This January meeting is a tradition, a meeting among researchers who, no matter how wide or diverse their membership becomes, devoutly think of one another as colleagues. Initially the Kenyans, Canadians, Americans, and Europeans came together around a single, small, overcrowded clinic in the middle of the city even before the onslaught of HIV/AIDS, and then discovered themselves uniquely positioned to take on a major role both in research around the new virus as well as in the enormous task of marshalling care for the thousands and ultimately millions in this region who would become infected by it. The collaboration, grown now to the more than 400 people who have signed up here, is described by seventy-two-year-old King Holmes as "generous and ecumenical." Holmes has come from Seattle, where he is director, since 1989, of the Center for AIDS and STDs at the University of Washington and founding chair of that university's department of global health. This collaboration "is something I could contrast, without naming names," he opines, "to other places where the groups are continually jealously fighting with each other rather than collaborating."

The context is public health: preventative health, epidemiology, control of this epidemic now into its second generation. The recently coined term "global health" recognizes at long last that the health of populations, especially with regard to infectious diseases, is no longer (if it ever was) a local question. The principle is that the health of every nation depends on the health of all others and this, as an esteemed *Lancet* journal panel noted more than a decade ago, "is not an empty piety, but an epidemiological fact."[1] The field of global health is also the landing place for people who spend their waking hours thinking about what are commonly called IDs, infectious diseases.

As we settle into the twenty-first century, it can be said that the *real* war of the worlds is a battle engaged not between organized societies and human or political terrorists, dramatic and tension-filled as those conflicts may be, but between human beings and microbes, the bacteria and viruses that occupy the vast unseen spaces both around us and within us. Microbes are by far the most abundant forms of life on earth, constituting some twenty-five times the total biomass of all animal life.[2] They are everywhere—in the air, the water, the soil, inside our bodies. The vast majority of the more than a million known types are harmless, in fact beneficial and essential to processes like digestion of food or decomposition of waste matter. But on the more sobering side, 1,415 are identified as capable of causing our death. This is the group that takes the attention of the infectious disease specialists.

Bacteria are free-living organisms containing a single chromosome and the ability to reproduce themselves. Viruses are something else, defined colourfully by the biologist awarded the Nobel Prize for medicine in 1960, Peter Medawar, as "a piece of nucleic acid surrounded by bad news."[3] Truly parasites, microbes, in order to survive, need hosts, something or somebody to live off. They are promiscuous and voracious in their appetite for ever-new hosts. To fulfill this need, they have developed a variety of means of getting around, as well as means to latch onto ever new and fertile hosts. Some viruses, like SARS, can be transmitted through the air, pushed by the force of a sneeze or a cough, or by simple breathing. Others, like the bubonic plague, which travelled on fleas, or malaria, which needs to pass through a mosquito, hitchhike from one subject to the next on the backs of "vectors." Some, like cholera and other gastroenteritis-causing microbes, are carried by fecal contamination in food and drinking water. Another group (syphilis, gonorrhea, HIV, and over thirty others) jump from one human to the next when people engage in sexual contact. Microbes vary in their virulence. In the case of poliomyelitis, the dreadful infection that persisted in the West right up to the middle of the last century, less than one in a hundred of those infected by the polio virus came down with the paralytic disease. Smallpox, by contrast, has regularly killed a third of those infected and scarred, blinded, or maimed the rest. With HIV, infection rates as a function of exposure have proven incredibly variable. Scientists such as Michael Oldstone gauge the risk overall as fairly low; approximately 5 percent of those exposed get infected.[4] The hazard per sex act is undoubtedly even lower, and the risks of infection as a function of exposure swing wildly under the sway of a myriad of influences.

For all of history, with the exception of the last 150 years, we humans and our ancestors have survived (sometimes barely) the onslaught of infectious diseases without the least understanding of their cause, and with virtually no effective treatments. Superstition, for most of our history, was as likely as not to rule the day. Occasionally, something resembling "science" was applied; Hippocrates, the Greek "father of modern medicine," importantly distinguished between those diseases that are *endemic*, that is, confined to doing their damage within a specific locale or neighbourhood, and those that are *epidemic*, that threaten to spread beyond that locale and into the wider world. But two thousand years would pass before his successors, physicians like Louis Pasteur and Robert Koch,[5] would develop and, more importantly, popularize the germ theory of infectious disease. It wasn't magic or God that brought plagues, but unclean water or sick people mingling with the rest of the population and sharing those invisible microbes. Meanwhile epidemics, the rapid spread of virulent diseases, plagued the world on a regular basis with kill numbers that put competing catastrophes such as wars, earthquakes, and tsunamis to shame. Extraordinary numbers died: 30 to 70 percent of Europe in the Black Death in the fourteenth century; 300 million in the twentieth century alone from smallpox; infinitely more killed by the influenza that followed the First World War in 1918–19 than died on the battlefields; 30 million dead and counting in our own time from HIV/AIDS.

Briefly, during the period of the discovery and perfection of the first vaccines and then the first antibiotics, all of which happened in little more than a century between the 1840s and the 1960s, or between the Crimean and Vietnam wars, what happened was a growing belief that the diseases that had ravaged the world could be—indeed, had been—tamed. Extraordinary accomplishments had certainly been registered. The mighty weapons of vaccines and antibiotics—antibiotics such as penicillin and sulpha drugs to kill bacterial infections, and vaccines to protect against viral ones—were unleashed. And these, combined with public sanitation, the concerted attack against perinatal mortality, the saving of greater numbers of both infants and birthing mothers at the time of childbirth, and greater protection of children in their first years of life literally changed the world, or certainly great parts of it. Epidemics were hit with increasingly standard strategies: vaccines to augment natural immunity, clean-up of stagnant water and open sewage to get rid of vectors, quarantines to isolate the infected. In 1967, nearing the end of that heady period, United States surgeon general William Stewart famously told the world that the book on infectious diseases could be closed.

Then, in the 1970s, something happened. New and sometimes lethal microbes began to emerge, surprising everybody, as they have done ever since, hitting us at the rate of around one a year with the frequency now apparently increasing.[6] What, everybody had to wonder, had happened, or, is happening? One explanatory factor is resistance to drugs on the part of exceedingly clever and ever-shifting microbes. Their mutated forms have now found ways to fight off the antibiotic drugs that had briefly threatened to obliterate them. A second factor is the arrival of new zoonotic viruses (H1N1, SARS, and HIV), that is, diseases that have jumped from animals to humans. This transition is not new, but has always happened; smallpox, for example, was probably originally a monkey pox. But each time it occurs it creates a new equilibrium. HIV, we now know, has been transferred to humans several times since the 1930s, likely from chimpanzee "bush meat," though it did not spread significantly until the 1970s.[7] A third factor is more rapid, more extensive, and more popular global travel along with changes in human behaviour. Global travel has always been a factor in the spread of diseases, transporting new infections to locations where the citizenry has no immunity. In the thirteenth century, diseases travelled with the crusaders and with traders to and from the Orient. In the fifteenth century, they accompanied the Spanish to the New World (the Spanish famously carried smallpox to devastate the Aboriginal inhabitants of the Americas while succumbing themselves to yellow fever, which they had not seen before). Now when great numbers of us travel both for business and pleasure at extraordinary rates, as well emigrate permanently, diseases—SARS, HIV, West Nile, drug-resistant tuberculosis, to name but a few—all too often travel with us.

What all this meant was that if you were a medical graduate in the late 1970s or 1980s you would find infectious diseases suddenly back on the menu as a challenging and honourable, not to mention potentially profitable, calling. After a hiatus of less than a generation, the world of the ID specialist has returned as a field with a growing cadre of experts and postings and an increasing cachet. "In the 1970s people were saying infectious diseases is a go-nowhere career—we're about to have it all under control," a young physician on the cusp of her career told me. "Well, we know that didn't happen." This young woman with a bright future is part of the next generation, which can once again get excited about infectious diseases and see it as a field of mission in bringing about a newly minted project of global health.

In 1968, at about the same time the U.S. surgeon general was declaring the battle against infectious diseases won, a young Canadian physician was returning home from graduate studies at the Universities of Maryland and Washington in that very field. The University of Washington was a world leader in infectious diseases research, and Allan Ronald, who had been there from 1965 to 1968 as a trainee, was excited by his experiences. Ronald was born on a farm near Portage la Prairie, Manitoba, into a deeply religious family out of which he was the first to head off to pursue higher education. When he came back to Winnipeg, he did not feel in sync with voices like Stewart's, but believed infectious diseases would continue to need strong academic leadership. His life's work, he thought, ought to be to try to replicate what he had encountered in Seattle. He decided he wanted to make his home province of Manitoba and the University of Manitoba a leader in the field. "Not that we would be Harvard or Johns Hopkins," he says referring to the large American universities with their vast endowments and iconic imprints, but there was, he believed, a place for smaller, regional players. The territory would benefit rather than suffer from decentralization. What was necessary was to understand how important the field was and to commit to it. While in Maryland, he had observed the Americans at the National Communicable Disease Center in Atlanta (which in 1970 would be renamed Centers for

Disease Control, the CDC) and its epidemiology branch under the leadership of Dr Alexander Langmuir. He had been deeply impressed; Langmuir had an unobstructed sense of mission, declaring bluntly that his mandate was to control infectious diseases first in the U.S. and then throughout the world. "This vision pervaded the whole institution," says Ronald, who got caught up with the idea of seeing something similar develop in Canada.

The University of Manitoba, in the late 1960s, was a provincial university almost a hundred years old, having been chartered in 1877. As the largest university in a small province, it needed in some sense to be all things to everybody. But if this forced it, in the opinion of some, to spread itself a bit thin, it had, right from the early days, always had a proud school of medicine, established in 1882.[8] Out of the Faculty of Medicine over the decades had come noteworthy contributions. In the 1930s and 1940s texts written by professors Swale Vincent on the study of secretion, A.T. Cameron on the biochemistry of medicine, and William Boyd on pathology all soared to prominence and "remained in use in their respective fields for many years."[9] Later, in the 1950s, Bruce Chown, Jack Bowmen, and Harry Medovy of the department of pediatrics were responsible for major breakthroughs in the diagnosis and treatment of Rh disease among newborn babies, an affliction that had caused roughly 10 percent of fetal and newborn deaths in North America. Not to be outdone, Henry Friesen, a 1958 graduate of the Faculty of Medicine, went off to McGill University and to post-graduate work in Boston, discovering, early in his career, the human hormone prolactin. He returned to Manitoba in the 1970s to head the department of physiology, where he continued research into human growth hormones. Later, as president of the Medical Research Council of Canada, he transformed the structure and funding of medical research in Canada.[10] In 1969, a high-profile and enduring enterprise was created under the auspices of the Faculty of Medicine by J.A. Hildes. The Northern Medical Unit (that would later bear Hildes's name) was set up to provide physician services to inhabitants of the remote north of Manitoba as well as undertaking research on the unique medical problems of northern (and Aboriginal) residents.[11]

It was to all of this that Ronald fixed his hopes and dreams.[12] However, that it should happen was not a given. Though he had been impressed by the University of Washington and by the foresight of Langmuir at the CDC, in Canada, at the time, you couldn't easily do the same thing. Powerful voices, like that of Douglas Cameron, head of medicine at McGill University and Montreal General Hospital, as well as president of the Royal College of Physicians and Surgeons of Canada, had latched on to the William Stewart line. "In Canada," Cameron said, "infectious diseases is an unnecessary discipline." For the moment, that opinion carried the day. There was no will in Ottawa, Ronald noted glumly, to invest in battling infectious diseases.

He had to wait a decade before the opportunity afforded itself to move his dream toward reality. By 1976, Ronald was a professor in the Faculty of Medicine and had been named head of the department of medical microbiology. This coincided, in 1975, with an outbreak in Winnipeg of a genital ulcer disease (GUD), also known as chancroid, caused by an organism named *Haemophilus ducreyi*. Ronald, who found himself in charge of responding, did two things. He set in motion the necessary lab work and became, with his research fellow Greg Hammond, the first to grow *H ducreyi* in the lab. Second, his team managed to treat and end the outbreak on the street, finding it to be transferred from prostitutes to clients in skid-row hotels. Word of their success got out—travelling quickly to the other side of the globe. Kenya had lots of sexually transmitted diseases, including chancroid, a fact only too well known to Ronald's counterpart there, the newly appointed chair of medical microbiology of the University of Nairobi, Herbert Nsanze. With an introduction engineered through the Geneva-based World Health Organization (WHO) in 1979, Nsanze approached Ronald at an international scientific conference: would he come to Nairobi to continue to study the epidemiology of chancroid? The Canadians would be welcome to do so if they brought their new laboratory technology with them and would agree to teach local scientists how to use it.

In January 1980, Ronald, accompanied by a researcher named Margaret Fast, arrived in Nairobi. At the time Margaret Fast was a thirty-five-year-old rural-Manitoba-born doctor doing tropical medicine training in England. She had no aversion to travel and had put in time over the years in various places around the globe, including Vietnam, where she met and married her husband. In late 1979, she heard about the job possibility in Nairobi, collecting samples and running the lab Ronald hoped to set up. Fast took the offer and in January she, her husband, and two small sons were off to Kenya.

In Kenya, the University of Nairobi was only eight years old and getting established. Nsanze, its head of microbiology, was ambitious and committed to having his department make a difference. He was thrilled to embrace the arriving Canadians, though the facilities he could offer were modest. He gave them six feet of lab space at the university and arranged that the research could be conducted out of something called the Special Treatment Clinic in the very centre of Nairobi, nick-named the Casino Clinic because of its proximity to the

Casino Hotel and operated by the city council. There they would care for men suffering from a variety of sexual diseases. More than one person described the place as a "hell hole"; every morning 600 to 800 patients would line up to be examined by one of the two or three doctors on staff. The Casino Clinic was run by an eccentric and some would say autocratic physician, Lourdes J. D'Costa. Fast's recollection of D'Costa was that he was "acerbic," which, compared to many accounts, was charitable. He was undeniably harsh. There are many recollections of him losing his temper and screaming at long queues of men suffering from painful ulcers to "go home, the clinic was closed, come back Monday." At other times he would tell them their suffering was their own fault. He did, though, allow the Canadian researchers access to his clinic, and the cumulative work of all of them together eventually rid Kenya of the scourge of chancroid.

D'Costa gave the Manitobans a small workspace and sent all the interesting cases their way. The whole business was run on a handshake and a shoestring. Margaret Fast became famous for "living like a Kenyan." She and her little family found a modest apartment about halfway between the lab at Kenyatta Hospital and the Casino Clinic. They bought a Volkswagen van in which to get around. "People kept stealing the headlights," she recalls, so her husband had steel mesh welded across them. "My husband had also befriended an Ethiopian fellow in Nairobi with no place to stay, so for awhile we let him sleep in the van," she told me. That served the double purpose of giving the homeless friend somewhere to lay his head and also provided theft protection for Fast's vehicle. Fast survived on a grant from a foundation, and Allan Ronald had his salary from the University of Manitoba, but everything else was cobbled together through contracts arranged with pharmaceutical companies to test various drugs on the patients. What would work best on the chancroid they encountered there? Ronald's wife Myrna was conscripted to help set up the clinic as a research unit. She recounts the struggle to get by on next to nothing: "Everything involved lining up, often for hours on end, whether it was to get proper papers to buy a vehicle, or to pay the electricity bill."

Things got off to a speedy start. Young researchers from around the world heard about the program and flew in: Peter Piot came from the Institute of Tropical Medicine in Antwerp, Belgium, and James Curran from the CDC in the United States. Curran, a year later, would get called back to the U.S. in response to reports of "weird cases of pneumonia" that needed urgent investigating. Ronald recalls a night in a restaurant with Curran and Peter Piot, the three of them puzzling over what might be causing these mysterious ailments. All too soon they would find out. Later, Curran's character would have a starring role in the movie about AIDS,

The Band Played On. Piot, who in 1976 had co-discovered the Ebola virus in what was then Zaire, would later spend thirteen years as head of UNAIDS, the United Nations' response to the HIV/AIDS epidemic. In 1981, he brought along other Belgian-trained physicians, Marie Laga, Leive Fransen, and Marleen Temmerman, who tracked syphilis among women in the public health clinics. And Ronald sent in his own most promising student, a young post-doctoral fellow named Frank Plummer, who arrived in January 1981 with his wife Carla. The WHO gave the enterprise its blessing and in 1983 designated the Nairobi project a Collaborating Centre for Sexually Transmitted Diseases, naming Herbert Nsanze the first director, followed in that position by J.O. Ndinya-Achola in 1984.

While specimen collection moved along, the laboratory work proved to be a frustration. "For the longest time we were not able to grow *H ducrei*," recalls Fast, who worked with a local technician, a Ugandan named Peter Karasira. To try to hurry things along Ronald brought in a young microbiologist from Winnipeg named Ian Maclean and, to Fast's relief, soon they were successfully growing the microbe. Maclean remembers being picked up by Ronald at Nairobi's airport, driven into the city with the car windows rolled down, and Ronald exclaiming: "Ian, take a deep breath, that's the smell of the Third World." To Maclean, the smell was that of exhaust fumes, overflowing sewage, and garbage.

Maclean spent three months in the lab, which he describes as an interesting though spare space donated by the department of medical microbiology in Kenyatta National Hospital. Outside the open windows, troops of convicts cut the grass with machete-like knives called *pangas* while watched over by a guard armed with a rifle. The lab consisted of a bench, a small incubator, microscopes, and a small centrifuge for spinning blood. There was no available supply of carbon dioxide, but "candle jars" served the purpose. "You put ten petri plates in," says Maclean, "then lit the candle. The candle would burn up the oxygen and that would be enough to produce about 5 percent CO_2, which organisms that cause chancroid and gonorrhoea require." The swabs, of course, were all from Casino Clinic. Every morning Frank Plummer would come with the samples and a set of hand-written log books in which every patient had a code number. After forty-eight hours in the candle jars, the researchers would be able to assess the results.

One side of the first lab was devoted to bacteriology, the other to serology, where syphilis was studied via rapid plasma reagin (RPR), an inexpensive test to determine exposure to syphilis. The first study was for a drug, Augmentin, a combination of amoxicillin plus clavulanic acid. Though the CDC recommended using penicillin against chancroid, the researchers in Kenya knew they could not do so because of an enzyme, beta-lactamase, that made the organism resistant to penicillin and penicillin-based drugs. The pharmaceutical company Beecham had discovered Augmentin, which contained amoxicillin plus clavulanic acid, a molecule that would bind the penicillin agent to the enzyme and prevent it from acting on the drug, and therefore amoxicillin could act on the organism and kill it.[13]

In early 1981, Margaret Fast and her young family finished their year and returned to North America. Twenty-nine-year-old Frank Plummer became her replacement. Plummer, likewise a product of small-town Manitoba, had specialized in internal medicine with an internship at the University of Southern California and a residency at the University of Manitoba, where he had worked under Ronald. In Nairobi, he continued with sample taking at Casino Clinic, an activity that little by little began to grow. Kenyans were hired to help out, including Ann Maingi, who was brought in to translate what was spoken in Swahili into English. Maingi quickly showed capabilities to do much more, and Myrna Ronald, a registered nurse, undertook to show her the ropes so that she could become administrator for the clinic. The young Kenyan, just out of high school, got a handle on the paperwork, specimen organization, planting cultures, and ordering supplies. She took to it all so effortlessly that she left to seek out proper lab training and still works in the project lab thirty years later. The project instituted a system of paying bus fare to the research subjects to make sure they would return for follow-up visits, critical both to their recovery and to systemized research. To get this arrangement working Carla Plummer marched every Monday morning from the clinic down to the local bank to obtain sacks of five- and ten-shilling (KSh) notes. In so doing, she had to negotiate River Road, one of the toughest streets in Nairobi, carrying enough cash to pay the week's clients.

Frank Plummer, ambitious, curious, and restless, soon cast his eye beyond the strict chancroid study by starting to quiz the men about their activities, especially their sexual encounters and the women they had been with when they contracted their infections. All stories led back to one place, the nearby Pumwani-Majengo shantytown and its thriving industry of sex workers. Working there, you didn't have to go far to come up against misery and challenges in need of fixing. While plotting how he might make inroads in the shantytown, Plummer turned his sights on the local maternity hospital. There, at a public hospital for the poorest of Nairobi's residents where each day dozens of babies were delivered, he encountered the neonatal conjunctivitis caused by gonorrhea and syphilis that resulted in far too many of those young babies losing their vision.

The response was to get more help. In short order, the collaboration and the research expanded. Robert Brunham, an infectious diseases physician and chlamydia specialist from Manitoba, started to pay visits. Elizabeth Ngugi, Kenya's deputy chief nursing officer, a senior official in the Ministry of Health, initiated a community-based program among female sex workers in Pumwani-Majengo. Frank Plummer took a research leave for a year at the CDC in Atlanta, but returned in 1984 to assume responsibilities for Canadian activities in Nairobi. In 1983 and 1984, efforts turned toward preventing infections in pregnancy and newborns, with initiatives set up in the maternity hospital that was just outside the shantytown. In 1985 the University of Washington joined the collaboration, and King Holmes, a friend of Ronald's from the 1960s, sent one of his most promising young fellows, Joan Kreiss. From Canada arrived a young pediatrician, Joann Embree, a Nova Scotia-born University of Manitoba trainee.

The Nairobi collaboration remained informal, almost ad hoc, until 1988, when it was formalized as a partnership between the departments of medical microbiology at the universities of Nairobi and Manitoba.[14] The first document, signed on January 11, 1988, outlined objectives of developing appropriate technology for prevention, diagnosis, and treatment of sexually transmitted diseases in developing countries while training workers and improving physical facilities to achieve those ends. The University of Nairobi wanted teaching programs strengthened in the fields of microbiology and infectious diseases, the chance to send the best of its students abroad for segments of their training, and improved laboratories and equipment. The University of Manitoba wanted to expand the opportunities for its students and faculty to work, learn, and do research in an atmosphere of international health. To those ends, both graduate students and faculty could look forward to travelling back and forth between Canada and Kenya and to being welcomed and given classrooms and labs when they landed.

CHAPTER TWO

The African Epidemic

I n 1984, Kenyan men were coming to the Casino Clinic in steady numbers loaded with infections and complaints. Frank Plummer, assisted now by Ann Maingi, had been asking them about their sexual activities, and the answers laid out a pattern. In case after case, the infected men had visited prostitutes, known locally as commercial sex workers, and overwhelmingly the location was identified as the nearby shantytown, Pumwani-Majengo. This densely populated enclave of tin-roofed shacks could stand as the quintessential definition of a shantytown. The community of cramped, overcrowded housing is almost totally bereft of services: no electricity, water only from standpipes, sewers running open and smelly. A stream struggling behind the houses at the bottom of a ravine is totally clogged with garbage. Few of the thousands of residents, many of them transients from other parts of Kenya or other countries, like nearby Tanzania or Uganda, possess basic items like identity papers, and nearly everybody is forced to cobble together their livings in what an economist might best spin as "an informal manner." A big part of this chaotic, informal economy is sex work: women entertaining clients in their meagre huts. Hundreds of women still do such work, three to ten clients per day, day after day after day.

The foreigners from Manitoba were not strangers to the shantytown. In 1983, after the departure of Margaret Fast and while Frank Plummer was away on his fellowship in the U.S., the only Canadian in Nairobi was a young doctor from Halifax doing his infectious diseases residency under the tutelage of Allan Ronald. David Haase soon made the acquaintance of Elizabeth Ngugi, someone with a deep interest in the welfare of the shantytown residents. Ngugi embraced the newly arrived outsider, and arranged for him to use a small clinic on the edge of the community to take care of sex workers. The building was one of three owned by Nairobi's city council. It was simple but sturdy, with a whitewashed facade. Nothing fancy, but in contrast to most construction in the shantytown, the glass was still in the windows, the floor remained uncracked, and the roof didn't leak. Haase was given the smallest of the three buildings, which would be used for a couple of years until a second, slightly larger building became available. Thirty years on, these clinics remain central to the project's operations. Then, as now, the clinic was a squash of four or five examining rooms ringing a crowded reception area. Through the open windows came an invasion of all the sights, sounds, and smells of the tumultuous neighbourhood—the market outside the clinic's front gates briskly selling everything from second-hand shoes (thousands of pairs) to T-shirts, fruits and vegetables, and even lace tablecloths. Every week, Haase would make his expedition not only to check the women and treat their sexually transmitted infections, but also to collect serum samples which he took back with him and placed in frozen storage.

A year later when Haase departed and Frank Plummer returned, Plummer decided he was going to gather a much larger cohort, maybe as many as 500 women, and by studying them get to the bottom of the infections that were being passed back and forth and ending up on the examining tables of the Casino Clinic. To make it happen, he approached the same public health official and community activist, Elizabeth Ngugi. Ngugi promptly offered to arrange a baraza, in shantytown parlance, a big party. There would be food, there would be jolliness, but the grand purpose behind it all would be addressing a local problem. One of those present was Leslie Slaney, then a young lab technician from Winnipeg. She explains how basically everybody gathered in what was an old community hall. "Elizabeth talked to the women about the infections and the risk and introduced the doctors from Canada who had come to help them. If they signed up, we would treat them for their infections." The baraza, as Ngugi, now a faculty member at the University of Nairobi and director of its Centre for HIV Prevention and Research, remembers it, was "the core of our being able to introduce ourselves. It was the way of saying, 'we are your friends. We are not your bosses, but your friends, together we can make you safer.' Friendship brings trust and a relationship." Two hundred women, she recalls, showed up. Discussion about the dangers of sexually transmitted diseases, however, did not include HIV. "We did not even know about AIDS," says Ngugi.

The baraza did its work. Great numbers of women from Pumwani-Majengo agreed to keep coming to the little clinic near the corner of their local market. "From then on we would see 150 women a week," says Leslie Slaney, "Wednesdays, Thursdays, and Friday morning."

Joan Kreiss, though young when it all happened, became a pivotal figure, wittingly or not, who turned AIDS research in a direction from which it could never be turned back. She had started her medical education in epidemiology at UCLA, which placed her in Los Angeles at the time, three years earlier, when the first cases of AIDS were recognized and reported. Armed with a natural curiosity, she decided to launch her research career by conducting a study of hemophiliacs already infected with the virus through transfusions of tainted blood to determine whether heterosexual transmission occurred between them and their spouses, and with what frequency. After finishing her fellowship at UCLA, she moved to Seattle to study infectious diseases under the tutelage of King Holmes. Determined to continue working on this new disease, HIV, she persuaded Holmes to send her to Nairobi. There, Plummer and Holmes tried to get her to help them with their studies on gonorrhea, but Kreiss had her heart set on HIV research and, learning that Belgian researchers had located cases of HIV in Rwanda, insisted on pursuing the new mysterious disease.[1] Holmes and Plummer relented. "She knew exactly what she wanted to do," Holmes remembers, "and the smartest thing I did was not stand in her way."

When she set to work, Kreiss wanted a subset of the women already frequenting the Majengo clinic, five each day, among whom she was going to look for HIV. She set up two cohorts, one with the Majengo women and then another with a group of sex workers downtown who were on the whole younger and of a higher social status. "Prostitutes in different settings had different kinds and nationalities of partners," she explains today as her rationale. "So I wanted to study women from a higher socioeconomic class setting." She selected a bar attached to a downtown tourist hotel and persuaded the proprietor to rent her a room to be used as a temporary clinic. Kreiss recounts an early visit to the bar one night in order to meet some of the women and see if they would be interested in participating in the study. The bar, called Buffalo Bill's, wanted you to believe you were in the American wild west, not Africa. Its "very distinctive and bizarre décor," Kreiss recalls, "lent a somewhat surreal quality to the whole endeavor."[2]

The research technique was to draw twenty-five millilitres of blood from each participant. Technologies designed to read what the samples showed were, at that time, rudimentary. Now, going on thirty years later, every clinic in Kenya can tell you your HIV status within fifteen minutes after the simple prick of a finger. In 1984, this was far from the case. A local lab technician at the Kenyan Medical Research Institute (KEMRI) was able to quantify T cell subset numbers in the samples, which was immensely useful. In the absence of a proper serological test, abnormalities in the T cell subsets were considered a useful surrogate marker for HIV infection, and seeing them gave the researchers some idea of what they were looking at. But getting a definitive result required a great deal more time and patience. The samples needed to be carried to America, to a lab at the NIH in Bethesda, Maryland, where the serum was tested for the antibody to HTLV-III. Then, for confirmation, they were submitted to something called the Western blot test. It took eight months for the official word to come back, and when it did, it was devastating. Of the sixty-four poorer sex workers from the Pumwani cohort, with an average age of twenty-nine years, 60 percent were HIV-positive. Of the twenty-nine women tested at the downtown bar, with an average age of twenty-four, 31 percent were HIV-positive. Eight percent of forty men from the Casino Clinic were positive, as was one person from the forty-two medical students and lab staff who were tested as a control. There could be no doubt: HIV was in Kenya.

"Everybody was totally shocked," says Frank Plummer. "Here we had HIV already infecting two-thirds of certain groups." "We knew," adds Allan Ronald, "that we were looking at an epidemic." Almost instantly, Plummer mapped out enlarged follow-up studies. One of them would be with a still larger group of commercial sex workers; the second promised to continue to follow women who were not infected with HIV in the first study to see if (and when) they might become HIV-positive. Their main aim was to isolate risk factors. Leaving no stone unturned, the researchers also went into the specimens collected by David Haase (with a kind of serendipitous foresight, even though he claims he did not consider HIV/AIDS when collecting the samples and barely knew about the disease at the time), had them tested, and discovered that in 1983 there was already a 4 percent infection rate, a rate that then jumped to 25 percent two years later.

The now commonly known story about the way human immunodeficiency virus (HIV) works is that it enters the cells of a host where it can persist unnoticed for a very long time. Damage develops slowly, stealthily breaking down the immunity of the patient. Actual illness can take a long time to set in, years in many cases, during which time the infected person shows few if any signs of poor health. In the end, though, the immune system collapses sufficiently that an opportunistic disease, often pneumonia or tuberculosis, moves in and the patient, not able to fight it off, succumbs. In the early 1980s, however, none of this was known. What the world was witnessing were eruptions in various places of a puzzling illness. In December of 1981, Michael Gottlieb and a group of colleagues at UCLA examined four homosexual males hospitalized for prolonged bouts of fever and multiple bacterial, fungal, and viral infections, all signs of a faulty immune system. All four developed *Pneumocystis carinii* pneumonia and one had a rare tumour, Kaposi's sarcoma. The doctors reported this puzzling phenomenon, which for a short time was labelled GRIDS, Gay Related Immune Deficiency Syndrome. But what appeared to be limited to gay men in America, in New York City and Los Angeles and San Francisco, was not limited to them at all, nor to America. That same year, Peter Piot recalls a stream of patients arriving from central Africa, the old Belgian colonial areas, to the Institute for Tropical Medicine in Antwerp, suffering from puzzling cases of infections. The arrivals were all wealthy Africans, senior army and government officials, well enough off to get themselves to the European hospital—where they died. "But we didn't know what it was they had," says Piot. "They had similar symptoms to what we were hearing from America, but there were both men and women, and the men insisted they had not had sex with other men."[3]

Neither were the American cases among gay men likely the first casualties of the infection. The first explosive epidemic is now believed to have occurred in the late 1970s in Kagera, a western province of Tanzania bordering Lake Victoria, from where it spread to next door Rwanda, Burundi, and southern Uganda. From there the virus is believed to have made its way east to the rest of Tanzania, to Kenya, south to Zambia, Malawi, and Zimbabwe, and then to the rest of the continent.[4] The first adequately documented report of an African outbreak came in 1984, when a Ugandan government official from the southern district of Rakai informed the Ministry of Health in Entebbe that young adults in the area were dying of a mysterious new disease that the locals called "Slim." He noted that the symptoms resembled those of AIDS, the disease that was killing homosexuals in the West.[5]

Attempts to definitively track down the origin of HIV/AIDS have proven an elusive mystery. Along the way, all manner of rumour, myth, and accusation have been levelled, little in the service of actual truth or knowledge, lots at the behest of politics and blame. The mystery was finally decoded to irrefutable and general satisfaction in 2006: HIV/AIDS did start in Africa as a zoonotic infection; contaminated blood from two simian (monkey) species contained the infectious agent that jumped the species barrier and entered humans who butchered the animals for food. The conclusion is that HIV-1 came from the African chimpanzee *Pan troglodytes* and HIV-2 from the Sooty mangabey somewhere around Kinshasa in the Democratic Republic of Congo, where the earliest known infection has now been unearthed, first documented in 1959.[6] As the epidemic unfolded, patients—like those seen by Gottlieb—appeared in the U.S., Europe, and Haiti infected, very likely, by sexual contact while travelling.

As far as its name is concerned, HIV/AIDS didn't get the name that finally stuck until the first scientific papers saw publication in 1983. Credit for using the term "Acquired Immunodeficiency Syndrome" goes to Luc Montagnier and Françoise Barré-Sinoussi, recognized in 2008 with the Nobel Prize for Medicine. Their work was carried out at the Institut Pasteur lab in France. A year later an American, Robert Gallo, published his findings that "retroviruses were a cause of AIDS." The internecine battle for the right to claim discovery has been waged off and on ever since, labelled by some as "the great Franco-American virus war."[7]

What was never in dispute from about 1983 onward was that HIV/AIDS was deadly and that it had the potential to be everywhere, a true epidemic. What is most critical when trying to understand HIV/AIDS, however, is to accept that *there is no single global HIV epidemic*, but rather a number of diverse epidemics. The worst of these, for a variety of reasons, has turned out to be in eastern and southern Africa. Several things differentiate the African epidemic from AIDS in other parts of the world. Firstly, it is "generalized." This means that transmission is sustained by sexual behaviour in the general population, as opposed to special sub-groups. It means that AIDS would spread even if programs for vulnerable groups were initiated that in its opposite, a concentrated epidemic, would work. This has made for very different challenges facing those who have confronted the epidemic in Africa. After watching the epidemic for almost twenty-five years, Richard Horton and Pam Das, in an editorial in the *Lancet* in 2008, posited that in a generalized epidemic like Africa's, the analysis demands greater focus on understanding how to fundamentally change societal norms of sexual behaviour. This is what had been learned: investments need to focus on promoting normative and social change to reduce multiple and concurrent partnerships, and on greatly increasing the availability of safe and affordable preventatives such as male circumcision services. The key research question: how to change fundamental community norms and to discourage multiple and concurrent partnerships.[8]

The other characteristic of the African epidemic was its rapid, unrecognized spread. Before long, the epidemic dominated life in eastern and southern Africa. The question often asked—though not even now adequately answered—is why the occurrence in Africa was so much higher than anywhere else in the world. The pieces of the puzzle manifested themselves through jumps in infection rates in various countries: in 1985 virtually no one in Botswana was HIV-positive; less than a decade later, by 1992, 10 percent of adults were infected, and by 2005 the number had rocketed to almost 40 percent. South Africa's infection rate rose from 5 percent in 1993 to 30 percent in 2005. By 2004, 42 percent of all adults in Swaziland were HIV-positive. Some declared that poverty was the common denominator and even that poverty was the cause of AIDS. Paula Treichler, a professor of communications research and women's studies at the University of Illinois, wrote in an essay on AIDS and the Third World, "In Africa, analysis of AIDS must inevitably confront questions of de-colonization, urbanization, modernization, poverty, endemic disease, and development."[9] True, but at the same time not so simple: all of Africa is poor, but not all of Africa has very high rates of HIV. Rates of HIV in the west of Africa stayed low. The overwhelming conclusion was narrowed down to this: HIV reaches very high levels only in areas where the sexual debut comes early, where there are lots of simultaneous sexual partnerships, lots of untreated STIs, lots of uncircumcised men, and no effective public health services.[10]

It took a while for many in the world to accept that heterosexual transmission was reliable enough to actually promote an epidemic like Africa was seeing. In the early days, what Michael Gottlieb confronted in Los Angeles and what Peter Piot witnessed in Antwerp looked like the same thing medically, but what didn't jibe was the information each of them had about the patients in front of them. So irrevocably was the new disease linked to gay, that is anal, sex in the minds of those looking at it that having any other perspectives proved difficult, at least during the early, critical months. The substantial difference between Africa and the rest of the world—that in much of eastern and southern Africa HIV is spread by something most people do, heterosexual sex—caused a stumbling block. As late as 1996, *Scientific American* magazine carried a much-read article by Australian anthropologists John C. and Pat Caldwell, expressing the common belief that "if a man and a woman are otherwise healthy except for the fact that one is HIV-positive, then in a single act of unprotected vaginal intercourse the chance of transmission from the man to the woman is one in 300 and from the woman to the man, possibly as low as one in 1,000."[11] This level of risk, they went on, contrasts sharply with the much greater likelihood of infection during unprotected anal intercourse or when sharing needles during drug use, or from a transfusion of infected blood, all the things driving the epidemic in the West. Yet, they had to admit, "despite our initial skepticism, evidence for the heterosexual epidemic in Africa is convincing. The most careful studies have shown that the infection rate among females is probably 1.2 times higher than the infection rate among males."[12] Not only did East Africa have a heterosexual epidemic, it was the only place in the world with a predominantly *female* epidemic.

WHAT MADE IT SO?

Why was HIV in Africa transmitted by heterosexuals while this did not happen to any great degree in Europe or North America? Tufts University historian Randall Packard and Harvard Medical School professor Paul Epstein raised two plausible theories. One was that AIDS had existed for a longer period of time in Africa than in the West and had therefore reached a different stage in its epidemiological history. The other had to do with unique aspects of African sexual behaviour: "higher levels of promiscuity or poly-partner sexual activities," they wrote, describing "the businessman or bureaucrat with a string of lovers, or the truck driver with sexual contacts across the map."[13]

In her book *The Invisible Cure, Africa, the West and the Fight against AIDS,* writer Helen Epstein pitted Africa's devastation against what the rest of the world experienced. The HIV rate in the United States never exceeded 1 percent, she noted: "In Russia and India, the figure also hovered around one percent. Even in Thailand with its thriving sex and drug trades, the national infection rate peaked at only around two percent in the early 1990s." She observed how at first some UN officials predicted that HIV would spread rapidly in the general population of Asia and eastern Europe, but though the virus had been present in those regions for decades, such extensive spread had never occurred. "Instead," she writes, "the virus remains confined to those with well-known risk factors such as prostitutes, intravenous drug users, and gay men who might have scores or even hundreds of partners a year." By contrast, "in East and southern Africa, virtually everyone is at high risk of HIV infection even though intravenous drug use is rare and few people have large numbers of sexual partners."[14]

Everybody, from academics to informed researcher-writers, came to believe that what was needed to solve the puzzle of Africa's spread was a better understanding of patterns of heterosexual sex unique to eastern and southern areas of that continent. Ultimately, one theory gained traction, and it had to do with a sexual sociology labelled "concurrency." Researched in Uganda by a University of Washington sociologist, Martina Morris, this theory suggested how sexual behaviour and cultural mores left people particularly open to the spread of the virus. It goes something like this: while a North American might have numerous sexual partners, the pattern by and large is to have them in sequence, ending one relationship before starting the next. In East Africa, more people were likely to have ongoing sexual relationships with more than one person simultaneously—or "concurrently." In Ugandan society, Morris found, the practice of maintaining an ongoing relationship with both a primary sexual partner and one or more secondary or more casual partners, simultaneously, over an extended period of time, was common enough to allow her to construct a plausible model.

Morris and a Dutch mathematician, Mirjam Kretzschmar, published their model, "A micro-simulation study of the effect of concurrent partnerships on the spread of HIV in Uganda" in 2000.[15] For poor Africans, as opposed to Westerners, though they may be no more (or even less) promiscuous, the interlocking sexual network that result from the concurrent practices creates a kind of HIV superhighway, linking people into a web of sexual relationships that can extend across huge regions. If one member contracts HIV, then everyone in the web is immediately placed at very high risk as well. This took a stab at explaining why so many African people—especially women—who are not promiscuous and who have had very few lifetime partners are nevertheless HIV-positive. The singular factor that made such behaviour dangerous was the period of overlap in relationships (in Uganda, 40 percent of men and 30 percent of women told Morris that at least two of their most recent relationships overlapped for several months or years) and the fact that HIV is always more potent for spread just after it has been newly acquired by a fresh host. While the HIV-positive person will transmit the virus on average only once in a hundred or so sex acts, the genetic "trick" of the virus that allows it to spread quickly through long-term concurrency networks is that it is most infectious during the first few weeks a person has been infected. During that time the infected person's blood teems with the virus. The conclusions in Uganda showed that "a recently infected person may be a hundred or even a thousand times more likely to transmit the virus than someone who has been infected for a few months or years."[16] This is known as the "viremic window" and explains also why the virus spreads so much more slowly in populations practising serial monogamy.

As would be confirmed over the next two decades, other things coalesced to create a kind of perfect storm. Public health systems (or the absence of them), for example, played a substantial role in how the epidemic progressed. Treating people's STIs, whether those be chancroid, genital ulcers, or herpes (HSV2), made a difference in HIV susceptibility. Not treating them, or not having the resources to treat them, resulted in higher susceptibility and higher rates of HIV. As seen in Morris's study, these concurrent sexual behaviour patterns were not completely straightforward—they could be complicated by multiple factors such as commercial sex, intergenerational sex, where an older man takes on a younger woman or even girl usually on the promise of financial support, and discordant couples, where one partner indulges in risky sex and the other doesn't. All these worked to push the AIDS epidemic in Africa forward.

The Caldwells, again, had noted differences between African and other societies in attitudes toward multiple partners. About traditional (and predominantly rural) sexual practices in Africa, they wrote: "infidelity might occasionally spark fights, punishment and, more rarely, marital dissolution, but it was never equated with sin and excoriated in the way that it was in traditional Western and Asian societies. Much good flowed from this permissive attitude; women were not suppressed and hidden, and girls had survival chances as great as their brothers'. But eventually these cultural traditions and attitudes did make the societies susceptible to attack by sexually related diseases."[17]

For its part, Uganda, where Morris did most of her work, experienced a "miracle" from about 1990 onward, with AIDS rates dropping (infection rates fell by about 70 percent between 1990 and 2001). It all had to do with what looked like an almost spontaneous behavioural change on the part of Ugandans, though examination showed there were both public policy and public education efforts behind it that went all the way up to the office of President Yoweri Museveni. The local groundswell was a homegrown campaign called "Zero Grazing" that was pushed by everybody from the president to local health educators and local pop stars. The outside world watched with fascination as it became clear partner reduction—more than even condom use—was the determining factor in reducing the risk of AIDS. Morris's hypothesis was proven true, at least in part.[18]

In Kenya, concurrent sexual practices were identified early on by researchers who decided to look at commercial sex workers and the kinds of clients with whom they were most likely to consort. In 1993, journalist Ted Conover published a long article in the *New Yorker* magazine entitled "Trucking Through the AIDS Belt."[19] It recounted weeks spent in the cabs of huge lorries with the drivers and the "turn boys" (drivers' helpers) hauling freight from Mombasa up through Kenya, around the Lake Victoria port of Mwanza in Tanzania, and through Rwanda. The drivers, away from home for weeks at a stretch, lived the life of truck stops, cheap hotels, and paid sex. The account provides some of the early information about habits and attitudes—how, for instance, condoms were available but expensive, and the prevalent myth that a man could cure his HIV infection by having sex with a virgin. The article also identified one of the early researchers of the spread of AIDS in East Africa, Job Bwayo of the University of Nairobi, who had opened a small clinic at Athi River east of Nairobi, where his early research identified that 27 percent of the drivers were HIV-positive.[20]

As the reality of HIV/AIDS became apparent, there had been a debate, Peter Piot recounts, among the members of the Nairobi collaboration about whether to put energy and resources into this new disease, or to concentrate on what they were already doing with good effect on known sexually transmitted diseases. In early 1986, members of the group including Frank Plummer, Joan Kreiss, Peter Piot, Allan Ronald, and King Holmes, gathered in Kisumu for a workshop ostensibly about opthalmium neonatorum, the infection that caused blindness in newborns. Stephen Moses, at the time a representative of the International Development Research Centre (IDRC), the Canadian Crown corporation that sponsored the meeting, was also present. He says that though the meeting was about opthalmium, "all the talk was about HIV. We realized the future was HIV; we couldn't keep people off the subject." Back in Nairobi, as Peter Piot tells it, "Frank Plummer argued that we needed to shift our attention to AIDS." So, as soon as the results started to come back from Joan Kreiss's samples, they did three things. First they attempted to sort out what this new information about an as yet novel—but deadly—disease would mean for how they provided care to the people who were coming to their tiny research posts. Second, they tried to pinpoint research strategies they ought to undertake to learn more about what they, and ostensibly the world, were up against. And third, they decided they could not and should not keep the information to themselves. The IDRC promptly stepped up to provide financing to help establish NARESA, the Network of AIDS Researchers of East and southern Africa.

Kreiss's findings were published in 1986 in the *New England Journal of Medicine* under the title "AIDS Virus Infection in Nairobi Prostitutes."[21] Almost immediately, the article was widely cited. The situation in Nairobi was now not only public, it was *very* public; the whole world knew. And while all the Kenyan colleagues who had been part of the clinic studies of the women and the lab work knew, now the Kenyan press and the Kenyan government also knew, and earlier felt singled out. A few months earlier, in November 1985, *New York Times* writer Lawrence Altman, after spending a month in Rwanda and Kenya, where he had become aware of Kreiss's at that point not yet published study, wrote an article that appeared on the front page of his newspaper. Under the headline "AIDS in Africa a Pattern of Mystery," Altman wrote how women and newborns seemed to be affected as much as were men and reported on the speculation that, though the first recognized cases were in the United States where 70 percent of sufferers were gay, the disease might have started in Africa.[22] A firestorm erupted. The article was carried globally in the *International Herald Tribune*, whose full shipment, when those papers arrived at Kenyatta International Airport, was confiscated by Kenyan officials. Altman had written into his story how paranoid African leadership was, and how the doctors he'd interviewed in Rwanda had insisted on not being identified. He quoted Peter Piot and Joan Kreiss's study, making the point that though no African country had as yet reported *any* cases to the WHO, there was certainly AIDS in Africa.

The storm should have been no surprise to anybody. AIDS was a mystery that few understood, a frightening disease with no proper explanation of its origin and no definitive projections of the harm it might wreak. Some in Africa were all too ready to label it a Western colonial plot, and their views got traction. The rumours that it was a disease of American gays was an explanation embraced by many in the African establishment, who clung to it mightily. Anything different, anything that placed either the origin or the epicentre of HIV/AIDS in Africa, would affect, for example, the immensely important tourism industry. The atmosphere in which AIDS was getting parlayed became chaotic and loaded with paranoia. *Medicus*, the official organ of the Kenyan Medical Association, tried to refute the "African origin" theory with its own hypothesis that tourists from around the world had introduced AIDS to Africa.[23] Again, the fact that AIDS killed people was bad enough, on top of that was the special shame of it being sexually transmitted, something addressed by Susan Sontag when she wrote that "infectious diseases to which sexual fault is attached always inspire fears of easy contagion and bizarre fantasies of transmission by non-venereal means in public places."[24]

Larry Gelmon was at the time a field officer for the IDRC, and he recollects the charged atmosphere over the next couple of years. "Both the Paris AIDS meeting in 1986 and the Washington AIDS conference in 1987 had a lot of controversy about HIV in Africa," he recalls. "The response in Africa became largely about who to blame; Kenyans blamed Tanzanians, who blamed Ugandans and so on. It was like the fifteenth century when people in Europe heatedly debated whether syphilis was the Italian disease or the French disease."

Throughout Africa, governments did not respond in concert, but in ways as different as night and day. As already noted, Uganda's government jumped to action fairly promptly, acknowledging the epidemic by 1988, and mounting public awareness campaigns about its dangers. South Africa, by contrast, while increasingly hard hit by the disease, remained preoccupied through the 1980s and 1990s with the fight against Apartheid and the transition to majority black rule, and then had the first decade of the twenty-first century taken over by "denialists" promoting dubious theories that denied even the connection between HIV and AIDS. Suspect treatments of beet root and wild honey were encouraged for the millions who were falling ill. Somewhere in the middle was Kenya, looking like it was in denial (although President Moi is rumoured to have warned his ministers early on about the risks of sexual misbehaviour) for almost fifteen years. Kenya would wait until 1999 before finally declaring HIV/AIDS a national disaster. It took another four years, to 2003, for President Mwai Kibaki to declare a "total war on AIDS."

The year 1986 was a long way from this. Not just caution, but paranoia and defensiveness ruled the day. After a reporter from the *Manchester Guardian* wrote a story about AIDS in Kenya, Peter Piot was summoned to the office of the Ministry of Health director of medical services, Wilfred Koinange. The purpose was to discuss whether Westerners like him and Plummer should be expelled from the country. "It was very intimidating," Piot recalls. "It wasn't just officials from the Health Ministry, but Security and Home Affairs. They said there was no AIDS in Kenya, and accused me of spreading false rumours. I had no right to do that, I was a guest in the country; they claimed there were serious indications I had violated laws." Piot had indeed spoken to a *Guardian* reporter, so he realized that his accusers were well-informed and that the fears about outsiders' phones being tapped or that they were being watched and followed had merit. He was made to wait for a full day in an anteroom of the ministry building while his fate was supposedly discussed in other offices. Finally officials came in to tell him he could stay in the country, "but I had to promise not to do it again."

What followed were a very difficult couple of years. Research wasn't stopped, but a chill enveloped everything. When Larry Gelmon came to Nairobi to visit his IDRC projects, he didn't leave his hotel room but had Plummer and Ronald come to him there because, he says, he was nervous to go out. "You had the feeling," he recounts, "that there were many in the government who didn't want to see a white face. I kept a low profile as a visiting donor. It's not unusual in this country [Kenya] for people who have run afoul of the government to get a knock on the door and have the GSU [government security] guys say, you've got an hour to pack your bags and get to the airport and out of the country. There was a climate of fear. The Canadians were here as the guests of the University of Nairobi and of the Kenyan government. They could just as easily lift our guest status." King Holmes recalls a visit to Kenya at around that time. "People were in denial and pissed at us," he says. He went out to dinner with a Kenyan academic, "an intelligent person whose firm position was either that the North Americans were fabricating the HIV epidemic, making it up, or, if it was real, it was a CIA plot to kill off Africa. It was really awkward."

As a young student, Joanne Embree believed her phone was tapped as she had no doubt Plummer's was. "When I went anywhere I didn't have to worry about being mugged," she recalls, "because I had the Kenyan secret service trundling along behind me. Every letter I sent home was opened." On some occasions she knew without any doubt that she was being observed. She recounts a dinner with University of Nairobi microbiology chair Hannington Pamba in a restaurant. The next day, Pamba had a visitor who made it clear that everything he had discussed with the foreign doctor was known. "Once it hit the press that there was HIV in Kenya," she says, "what the Kenyans feared they were looking at was a bunch of uncontrolled university professors from another country whose goal is science—and personal advancement in science—and who are not Kenyan."

All too soon, there was trouble again. This time it stemmed from research Plummer had undertaken as part of the first steps to determine the implications of the epidemic and how both science and their clinical work might play a role in identifying ways to contain it. An early observation was that widely used oral contraceptives made sex workers more susceptible to the virus, a highly controversial claim, to say the least. One argument was the obvious one: condoms were promptly identified as a prevention of HIV spread, and oral contraception worked against the use of condoms. But the pill, likewise, was determined to upset hormonal balance, as much as doubling the risk of infection. Though the information was not published until 1990,[25] Plummer spoke about it in a speech at the 1987 Third International AIDS Conference in Washington. There it understandably caused a sizable stir that then spilled out beyond the meeting's doors. Again, Altman of the *New York Times* wrote an article; the *Daily Nation*, the national newspaper of Kenya, picked it up, and back there, all hell broke loose. In a country and a continent where huge amounts of donor dollars and public policy had finally come round to population control through family planning, both the Kenyan government and the family-planning establishment were furious and thought Plummer irresponsible.

More directly, the response to Plummer's findings threatened his continued work in Kenya. He held local positions as a visiting professor at the University of Nairobi as well as at KEMRI. One morning he arrived at work to find his position at the latter suddenly revoked. It took action by Elizabeth Ngugi to save him from being expelled from the country. Ngugi went as high up in the chain of command as she could in the Ministry of Health, to the same official who had threatened to deport Peter Piot. She confronted him about the pressures on Plummer and tried to deflect any suggestion there was any motive beyond a search for truth. "I told him, this is not him [Plummer], this is science." Her pleas succeeded in keeping the Canadians in Kenya, but likewise laid down for at least some in the government the premise that scientific truth would be the only real useful weapon against the epidemic.

CHAPTER THREE

Educating Around AIDS

T here may have been confusion and even wilful denial at the official national level, but in Kenya, indeed in all East and southern Africa, those at street level quickly started to realize that AIDS was a catastrophe without foreseeable limits. Deaths began to mount, there was no cure, strategies at control were haphazard and weak. The disease was killing off not the old and feeble—like epidemics usually do—but the young and virile, those in their middle age, those who were sexually active. Its victims were the workforce of the country and the parents of the nation's young children. The numbers of those orphaned by AIDS started to grow, soon to become an avalanche. The questions in everybody's minds were frightening ones. What was AIDS? How did it spread? How could it be managed? If the terrifying disease was called HIV/AIDS, why were people dying of other things, like pneumonia and tuberculosis? Nobody had ready answers, not governments, not the media, not even scientists. The uncertainties generated by this cloud quickly settling over vast parts of Africa were disturbing everyone.

Not only international health agencies, but international aid organizations, took notice. Their response took some time to develop, but eventually it did. In 1989, the Canadian International Development Agency (CIDA) sent a consultant to Kenya to investigate how it might support a workable HIV/AIDS prevention initiative. Foreign aid agencies had begun to realize that HIV/AIDS was not just a health issue, but a major development issue. If the disease was not corralled and if it continued to decimate the educated workforce, it would affect national and even regional economies, turning back decades of material progress. The traditional foreign aid establishment had been slowly coming round to this sobering understanding. The American USAID would eventually spend $7 billion on the AIDS pandemic, but this was the early days of thinking in this manner, and this was the Canadian response.[1] "The human and social costs in certain settings are already or will soon be enormous," the consultant concluded. "The disease affects people in their most productive years, and is now threatening the next generation. AIDS also disproportionately affects Africa's skilled and educated classes."[2]

That CIDA was at last showing this interest was thanks in no small part to the lobbying of the Canadians in the Nairobi project, and a payoff for months and months of their efforts. For years, as they struggled to find the necessary funds for their expanding list of investigations, clinical interventions, and re-searches, they had gone to CIDA and been perplexed that they were continuous-ly rebuffed. The agency that managed 80 percent of Canada's almost $3 billion of foreign aid responded over and over that it could only finance development, not research. Finally, in early 1989, Frank Plummer and Allan Ronald made a trip to Ottawa where, at CIDA headquarters, they secured a meeting with a man named Steven Simon, the lead medical staffer. If they couldn't get support for medical research, they asked, what about help carrying out a vast project of public education and preparedness to confront the expanding epidemic? They laid out a plan that specified what they might do: develop protocols for diagno-sis and treatment of STDs as well as counselling protocols; upgrade laboratory skills in both rural and urban parts of Kenya and develop field tests and more appropriate diagnostic techniques to improve lab diagnosis of STDs. They pro-posed ideas about ways to target high-risk groups, which at the time everybody agreed were truck drivers and sex workers and their clients, and also ways to as-sess appropriate and effective plans to motivate behavioural changes in both the target groups and the population at large. Then they waited. It was a tall order and a big challenge. The CIDA official had listened carefully, but "we couldn't tell what he was thinking," Plummer remembers. "This work," he pronounced, "must be supported."

The government of Kenya had been notoriously slow—even reluctant—to admit that HIV/AIDS was a problem. It had, nonetheless, convened a multi-agency task force called the National AIDS Control Programme (NACP). What it wanted was foreign donor funding to help this program do its work. Robert Cushman, the consultant CIDA sent to survey the scene, however, had some misgivings. He noted that NACP had spent the entire year of 1989, "getting its own house in order." But on the other hand he was impressed that the Manitoba/ Nairobi STD research group could be counted on to be well organized and inno-vative. On his return to Canada he sent a letter to Allan Ronald in April of 1989 inviting a proposal to do what he and Frank Plummer had described to Steven

Simon in Ottawa, expand AIDS control in Kenya. "This," he stated, "now puts the ball firmly in your court for proposal development."[3]

Finally settled, the stated objectives of the new venture were to strengthen the provision of health services with respect to STDs and HIV/AIDS at health facilities in several field sites throughout Kenya. Local health workers would be trained to both diagnose and more effectively treat all kinds of sexually trans-mitted diseases. A main objective was to decentralize STD-related health ser-vice delivery, bringing it out to the countryside where people lived. They were also to train health workers and provide drugs, as well as design, implement, and evaluate community-based health educational, promotional, and counsel-ling programs that focussed on high-risk groups. What they were up against, they knew, were formidable gaps in the current state of things: inadequate train-ing of existing staff across Kenya, inefficient deployment of staff, high patient loads, lack of supportive supervision, inadequate referral mechanisms, shortag-es of clinical supplies and drugs, and inadequate record keeping. They realized that it was important to institute community-based peer education programs for women who sell sex and their clients, as well as for out-of-school youth and other vulnerable groups. They needed to promote less risky sexual behaviour and wider use of condoms across vast swaths of Kenyan society.

The result of the proposal they put together was a $3.1 million grant. The project, entitled "Strengthening STD/AIDS Control in Kenya," began in No-vember 1990 with the understanding being that after five years it could be re-newed. Now they needed staff to direct it, and in this they got lucky. Stephen Moses, who had come to Nairobi as the IDRC's regional representative, loved being in Kenya and let the Manitobans he encountered regularly through his IDRC work know that he would be happy to join their work. Moses was hired as the program's director. For the Kenyan side, they got one of the most dedicated public education officials anywhere, Elizabeth Ngugi.

Need for such a far-reaching program as this was self-evident; passion for it came from a deeply invested participant. Ngugi's entire philosophy, first as a nurse and then a public health official, was centred around the dignity of ordi-nary Kenyan people, even (or especially) those at the bottom of the socio-eco-nomic heap. She reserved a special place in her heart for those whose lives were the hardest, like the shantytown sex workers existing day to day, often without proper papers and the basic civil rights those conferred. "Human beings want to be valued for who they are," was Ngugi's operational mantra, repeated over and over. This meant progress of any sort could only be made by taking people into your confidence as partners, where you respected their views and worked to fulfill *their* agendas. "You need to work within their decision making mechanism, otherwise, forget it," she said. "You have to come to them and say 'we have a problem.'" The implication being that the problem was not their problem alone, but one that was shared.

Defining the problem of AIDS was a huge challenge. For uneducated or superstitious Kenyans, the onslaught of AIDS was comprehensible only in terms of consigning it to some kind of evil that had befallen them through witchcraft. To a good many, this explanation made as much sense as the explanations scientists were offering. The scientists too could only explain AIDS as a mystery that had come upon people in all walks of life and was afflicting them for the most abstract of reasons—you couldn't see a virus, you couldn't see it enter your bloodstream, you couldn't see it do its work. Those known to be infected were told they had a disease and that they would likely die from it. But for the time being they felt okay, not yet sick. Then they started to lose weight and become thin, which played into the witchcraft theories, because that's what a witch's spell could do to you. For a great majority of Kenyans, uneducated and struggling with so many different aspects of their lives, Ngugi knew that coming around on AIDS was going to be a process that took time. "Eventually they were seeing sickness and that made it more real to them," she said. "Seeing is believing." But it was a very difficult process to get to the point of believing.

Telling the women in the shantytown the disease was related to sex demanded even more of those women in response. To begin with, they were skeptical of the foreign scientists. How did the scientists know that this was so, they would ask? Some were truly suspicious, saying things like, "you don't know, you must be hiding something." Once they got to the point of believing it was a sexual disease, however, they were able to take control of it. They bought into the program, and the idea of preventive measures, especially condoms, made sense to them. In all this, Ngugi saw herself as something akin to a mother hen, an all-over-seeing presence with commensurate power and authority. She liked the image. "I'm a mother of sex workers," she said, "and people listen to their mother." Her dream was to take the message she had started with the baraza in the Majengo shantytown half a decade earlier to the whole of the country. A new grant allowed her to investigate four locations, including the agricultural towns of Nakuru and Thika, well away from the capital, where she hoped to replicate what had been started in microcosm in the Pumwani-Majengo shantytown of Nairobi. She would train health workers to work with sex workers, take care of the sick, and carry on the explanation of AIDS and the actions needed to prevent its spread. Over a decade and a half these projects would, in the end, help mobilize 15,000 to 20,000 sex workers to fight the spread of AIDS.

I once spent a day with Elizabeth Ngugi, having asked her to take me into her world. It was a world where she looked in on the sick and the dying, along with trying to educate the well and the living. We agreed to meet early on a Saturday morning at the edge of Nairobi's downtown. When she showed up, Ngugi was not alone; with her was a woman named Bernadette, the chairperson of a committee Ngugi had helped the sex workers put together to forward their interests. Bernadette smiled crisply. Dressed like a no-nonsense church woman and carrying a voluminous handbag, she was very much into her role as chairperson. I joined the two of them in Ngugi's vehicle and we headed into the middle of the city, ending on a street of commercial stores selling things like electrical appliances and auto parts, all the dusty unadorned components of construction and service businesses. Ngugi pulled up in front of a whitewashed building with a sagging green awning and a smudged sign: New Aden Hotel. "Come with me," she said, clambering out of her van. The director of community health for Kenya, wrapped in traditional dress, a colourful ground-length print with matching fabric folded around her head, West Africa style, headed for the front door past a beer vendor and a clot of loitering men. It was then that both I and the men noticed what she held in her hand: two pieces of wood, one light blond, possibly pine, the other dark ebony, about eight inches long, shaped and polished to a smooth sheen. Wooden penises. When she saw us looking, she laughed.

Inside, the hallways were gloomy as night. Up we went, three flights, at every landing stopping to exchange enthusiastic greetings with the people who emerged as if on cue from the doorways of the rooms, grinning women not to mention the odd bamboozled-looking man. Finally we reached the top, where an open door showed into a small room, the kind of low-end hotel suite that would never be rented by a foreigner. Seated on the sagging bed and two hardback chairs were four women, all of them commercial sex workers and all of them very large. Ngugi and Bernadette pushed in. Like a practised show host, the doctor leaned forward, flourishing, like a pair of chopsticks, the two penises. From her bag she pulled a fistful of shiny foil packets. "Now," she said in her heavily accented English, "what we are going to undertake is a demonstration with a group of women who work out of this hotel. Just to review what they know about condom use." The largest of the women, Alice, squeezed incongruously into an orange miniskirt, took the light-coloured pine stick and one of the condoms. The ebony rod was grasped by Florence, a crinkly-faced older woman. The sound of tearing could be heard as the foil encasing the condoms was ripped open. Though nobody could say what the statistics were among all Kenyans in general, condom use among sex workers in Nairobi, Ngugi said, had risen to 75 percent. Three-quarters of sex worker women used condoms three-quarters of the time, or some variant of that pattern. This was thanks to relentless public education, posters everywhere, including bars, and one-on-one instruction such as the lesson happening that afternoon.

It also was a result of a huge supply of condoms arriving as part of the foreign aid programs of North American and European nations. Condom supply was part and parcel of almost all aid packages and HIV/AIDS strategies; the Strengthening STD/AIDS Control in Kenya program handed out condoms at every opportunity, hundreds of thousands in total. Yet 75 percent use among this highest of risk groups seemed hardly good enough. In all the strategies around HIV/AIDS, one would have thought simple prevention should be the easiest, the cheapest, the most potentially fruitful. If ever there was a disease that was easier to prevent than to cure it was AIDS, yet, in a country with at least a 10 percent rate of infection, prevention was obviously not working very well.

The major culprits, almost every woman I spoke to in Kenya told me, were the men. "The customers," the sex workers reported, "will pay more for no condom." Despite all the information so chillingly available, men still blindly insisted on taking their chances. And men still liked a lot of sex. Kenyans, I'd long since learned, could not be conveniently boxed into a single monolithic cultural category; it was much more complicated than that. Tribal customs entered into it, as did levels of education and levels of adoption of Western-influenced urbanization and modernity. Everywhere could be found pockets of conservative communities, both traditional and Christian. But there was also a much more relaxed and recreational attitude toward sex than exists in general Western culture. In the view of not all but certainly many Kenyans, the right for an African man to have multiple partners might as well have been enshrined in the constitution. One evening I got into a conversation with a young fellow not yet out of his twenties. If education was a measure, this young man had to be aware of things for he had a university degree and a job with the government. But when we got around to discussing sex he told me bluntly, "A man who makes love to only one woman is not a real man." When I raised the matter of AIDS he looked at me as if I was truly wearisome. Sighing deeply, he marshalled his argument. "I might die from AIDS, it is true," he said. "But in the time it takes for that to happen I might also die in a shooting, a traffic accident, a war, or of some other disease." Life was a lottery and he would take his chances.[4]

We then headed off to the second appointment of our afternoon, a shanty-town on the opposite side of the city from Pumwani. We proceeded through the usual rigmarole, parking our vehicle then treading through a push of people and the stench of the litter-filled road toward the hut of a woman Elizabeth wanted to look in on. Turning down a narrow pathway between mud walls, she eventually pulled back a curtain masking a doorway. Inside was a skinny, near emaciated creature in bare feet and a rag dress—Jennifer, a sex worker in the late stages of AIDS. The rainy season was just commencing, and all the concerns I had every time I saw the architecture of the shantytowns would soon come to fruition. In the rain the night before a section of the mud wall outside Jennifer's hut had collapsed in a heap, exposing the crude sticks that served as lathwork. Even inside the hut, the packed mud of the floor stuck to your shoes. The anti-retroviral therapies that would have saved this woman's life were still almost a decade in the future. All that stared her in the face was a miserable death.

Elizabeth and Bernadette squeezed themselves onto the lumpy, damp pillows next to Jennifer. Outside, a few of the curious gathered round to peer in the doorway. Elizabeth wanted me to meet the children. Jennifer had six, so one of the women from outside was sent scurrying off to round them up. Elizabeth took a look at Jennifer and attempted to start a conversation, in large part for my benefit. She began to question and then explain the sick woman's symptoms. "She has chills, she has fevers, she has severe headaches," she said. With each description, Jennifer nodded her head weakly and looked ever more miserable. Many were the days when she could do nothing but doze. She had made her living as a commercial sex worker, and though it was terrifying to consider how long into her illness she might have continued to work, it was unrealistic to think that she would not have done so. But certainly there was no living to be made now. The miserable end was upon her, and her only hope to mitigate anything about it was seated on the bed beside her. "We are here," Ngugi pronounced firmly as if sermonizing to the whole world, "because we have to organize to look after the children. We have to make certain Jennifer gets what she needs." Throughout the shantytowns, as one by one women became ill, she and Bernadette were organizing care-giving cooperatives. Jennifer obviously needed a lot of help. The woman who had gone to fetch her children returned, having rounded up four out of the six. Their bewildered faces appeared in the doorway while in between them pushed a mangy dog.

This was the context into which the Kenya STD/AIDS Control Project needed to make inroads. Two years on, the program appeared to be going well. A monitoring report by CIDA in 1992 stated, "The (program) is judged to be largely successful and on course, and all involved are to be commended."[5] By then, sites out of which education and support would be offered had been opened in Nairobi and Nakuru, while staff were being trained for a second Nairobi location and an office in the northern town of Thika. The primary groups the program had targeted—sex workers, out-of-school youth, as well as school children, teachers, and parents—were all deeply engaged. Relationships with both central and local governments were judged to be on a good footing.

Still, the project required patience and attention to myriad details. A step forward would frequently be countered by something that went in the other direction. In his October 1992 report, Stephen Moses observed that the Nairobi city council had decided to levy user fees at its clinics. This attempt to raise money was having the predictable deleterious effect on patients with sexually transmitted diseases. Numbers of those showing up for attention had dropped significantly. After protests, the council reduced the user fees to a flat 50 KSh (about 65 cents) for STD patients, with no additional charges for drugs or lab work, and 10 KSh for gonorrhea treatments. Anything, though, that worked to discourage patients from going for medical attention was considered counterproductive to the objectives of fighting the epidemic. The Nairboi collaboration had, by this point, embraced the premise that treating any STD as promptly as possible was a crucial strategy in preventing HIV infections. It was also upsetting to the researchers that the sexual partners of STD patients were charged the user fee, something that worked against their willingness to come forward and adversely affected the program's goals of tracking the paths of infections. Moses also noted ruefully that "the funds generated by the out-patient user charge policy have not made their way to the City Health Department, but have remained in the City Treasury."[6]

This is how it went for the next fourteen years: obstacles along the way, but general progress. Seemingly endless meetings, training sessions, review sessions, and patience gradually pushed HIV/AIDS awareness to where it needed to be, on the front burner of Kenyan culture. The program was judged successful and its funding and mandate renewed twice over. "We were among the pioneers in setting up such programs," recounts Moses. In Kenya, the project worked to become more accessible, moving away from the highly centralized referral centres that were very difficult to access and had a lot of problems. Among these problems, says Moses, were "the stigmas attached to going in the first place, and then long line-ups when you got there." All was achieved with a Kenyan staff of about fifteen, who operated out of existing municipal council health clinics in a variety of centres across the country.[7]

However, because this was an arm of foreign aid, and because foreign aid inevitably has a political dimension to it, long-term security of funding was always chancy. How deep were both the pockets and the commitment of foreign taxpayers? Could the rich side of the world sustain the awe-inspiring levels of support Africa needed in its AIDS battle over ten, twenty, thirty years, and longer? The project suffered a big bump when CIDA underwent a change in its mandate back home. In the early 1990s the government in Canada changed and the new administration of Prime Minister Jean Chrétien and Finance Minister Paul Martin took a knife to the federal deficit. No department or bureau or program escaped re-evaluation, including foreign aid. For a few urgent weeks it looked as though CIDA's Africa programs—including the Kenyan one—would all end. A period of furious lobbying ensued. In Nairobi, Stephen Moses, Kelly Macdonald, and all other relevant personnel gathered night after night at Frank Plummer's house to organize overtures to everybody, from the country CIDA coordinator to Kenyan members of parliament to officers at the Canadian High Commission. They persuaded the new Canadian high commissioner to Kenya, a woman named Lucy Edwards, to pay a visit to their lab and clinics. She did so and immediately turned into a supporter, telling the researchers they needed to keep fighting. In Winnipeg and Ottawa, everybody with a pen wrote a letter and everybody with a voice was put on the phone. Bob Brunham, by then head of medical microbiology at the University of Manitoba, wrote to Lloyd Axworthy, Manitoba's senior cabinet minister in the Chrétien government, "several times." Allan Ronald asked high-profile academics such as Mark Wainberg, renowned AIDS researcher at McGill University and soon-to-be president of the International AIDS Society, to weigh in. In the end, their protestations prevailed, persuading the Canadian government to a change of heart that would allow the project to continue. It was the only CIDA project in Africa permitted to do so.[8]

Less than a decade later, by 2004, the project was winding down. In part, this was a testament to a growing Kenyan organizational expertise. The idea all along had been that innovations the Canadians had made should eventually become formalized and institutionalized, largely under the umbrella of the University of Nairobi. The Kenyan government, by this time, had streamlined its country-wide oversight into the National AIDS Control Council, which became a bridge between an inter-agency coordinating committee and—as UNAIDS had then mandated for every country to centralize HIV control—the office of the president. At the same time, the College of Health Sciences set the wheels in motion to create the University of Nairobi Institute for Tropical and Infectious Diseases (UNITID) and the Centre for HIV Prevention and Research. The program would not end easily, however. Challenges with its funder back in Canada persisted to the very end. What it had survived in the threatened funding cuts of 1996, it didn't escape in 2004 (see Chapter 9), when CIDA withdrew financing almost a year before the end of the contractual term.

CHAPTER FOUR

Research Strategies

A fter the 1985 study on HIV infection among Kenyan sex workers, the Manitobans and their colleagues from the University of Nairobi and the other universities in the U.S. and Belgium scrambled to roll out research strategies. They would expand their investigations with the new mothers they had under their care at the Pumwani Maternity Hospital to see if they could determine if and how HIV might be transferred from an infected mother to a fetus or newborn child. Then they negotiated with the council in the Pumwani-Majengo shantytown to continue working in the small free-standing clinics where they could follow female sex workers. In return for the women permitting themselves to be tested for HIV and giving up samples of their blood at regular intervals, they and their children would receive general health care. The researchers likewise strategized to follow up on a question that kept bugging Plummer, who was still seeing the patients with genital ulcers at the Casino Clinic: could there be a connection between STDs of all sorts and susceptibility to HIV infection?

AIDS had struck close to home. One of their own, a young Uganda-born lab technician who had helped Margaret Fast set up her research when she first arrived in the country, Peter Karasira, discovered that he was ill. Over months, his colleagues watched his health deteriorate, and then he died. If anything was needed to make all their work seem more urgent, this sad event certainly registered with everyone.[1] Kenyans at the ground level of the project dug in. From the beginning they had been deeply involved, partly because of the terms of the collaboration agreement, partly out of necessity. The sex-worker clinic in Majengo was overseen by Kenyan doctors, the first being Michael Gakinya, followed by Omu Anzala, Joshua Kimani, and Ephantus Njagi. Equally critical to making it really work were the nurses. One of these was Jane Kamene, who, when she was "young and green," as she puts it, had substituted for her sister-in-law, Ann

Maingi, when she took a maternity leave from duties at the Casino Clinic. That was 1983, and Kamene never left the project. When the sex-worker clinic opened, she became nurse there. For the next twenty-eight years and counting, her morning routine consisted of leaving her home and child before 7 a.m., joining the rest of the staff at the lab at the University of Nairobi Medical School at Kenyatta National Hospital for an early morning cup of tea, then gathering supplies as well as any special instructions for the day and climbing into the project van for the journey across the city. Squeezing in alongside her would be a revolving cast of clinicians, nurses, foreign medical students, and assorted visitors.

It was quite a trip, especially for any visitor fresh to Kenya. The expedition wended through the full variety of Nairobi's morning; whizzing under the green suburban canopy until, rounding a corner, it was abruptly halted by a traffic jam of the sort that can only materialize in Nairobi, a choke of fume-emitting vehicles penned in by hand-drawn carts and weaving pedestrians. A clever driver could find a way out by shortcutting through a petrol station or along a back lane and suddenly be on his way again, passing the hand-drawn carts and shiny Mercedes limousines alike until, once again, the streets narrowed and the lumbering lorries and pedestrian crowds of the poorer parts of the city ground everything back to a crawl. There was a series of drivers serving the project, but the main one for many hundreds of these early morning journeys was a taciturn though sharply alert man named Daniel N'gang Mukuria, affectionately known as "Mr D." Everybody had their supplies: Jane Kamene and the other nurses would have their boxes containing syringes, plates, and medications, whatever the agenda of the day demanded. Mr D, for his part, carried with him a couple of large jars of milk from the cow he kept tethered behind the house where he lived. His moonlight activity was to sell his milk to shantytown customers.

Record keeping was important in the short run, but proved to be infinitely more so in the long term. It was Jane Kamene who started to maintain a book into which, in order of enrolment, she entered the names of all the women who signed up for care and research at the sex-worker clinic. Each was given a number, starting with 001. Dates of enrolment and places of birth were entered as, sadly and all too often, were dates of death. In the fall of 2004, Jane brought out the book to show me that out of the 600 names registered, 152 had died. The book, black with a red binding, had by then been bleakly titled "Death Registry" and was a record not only of hope and research, but of the toll of HIV/AIDS.

After dropping off everybody who needed to be at the Majengo clinic, Mr D's job was (and still is) to steer his well-worn van back through the crowded alleyways of the shantytown, past the shoe-sellers and pineapple-loaded wheelbar-rows, and then get round the corner to the Pumwani Maternity Hospital. There he dropped off more staff along with the daily supplies for a different type of research and care—this with mothers and their newborns. The rationale for the work in the Majengo clinic was to keep tabs on sex workers, treat their ailments, and try to learn something from the patterns of their HIV infections. At the maternity hospital, the project was to learn if, how, and maybe why the infection travelled from mother to child.

Research with the sex workers yielded increasing volumes of information. In the June 1987 issue of the *Journal of Infectious Diseases*, Peter Piot and Frank Plummer reported how they had been able to track AIDS virus infections in Nairobi populations.[2] They had studied 446 sex workers in 1985, finding 61 per-cent of them to be HIV-positive. They then learned more about their subjects and determined that the sex workers who were HIV-positive, as well as any women with sexually transmitted diseases, tended to have more sex partners as well as a higher prevalence of gonorrhea. Conversely, of the women with STDs, significantly more who turned out to be HIV-positive also practised prostitu-tion. They discovered, as well, by asking the men and pregnant women with STDs where they had come from, that those who were born in the most western region of Kenya, near the Ugandan and Rwandan borders, were more likely to have the antibody to HIV than groups from other geographic areas. This meant they'd been exposed to HIV, even if they had not contracted it. Through glean-ing information like this, they were able to start to date and pinpoint the geogra-phy of the epidemic. "Our results," they wrote, "indicate that the AIDS virus was recently introduced into Kenya, that HIV can rapidly disseminate in a high-risk group of heterosexuals, and that female sex workers and their clients may have significantly contributed to the spread of the virus."

Two more Canadians from the University of Manitoba, Neil Simonsen and William Cameron, publishing their findings in the *New England Journal of Med-icine* in 1988, determined that the thirty-five HIV-positive men out of the 340 they studied had contracted their infection through heterosexual rather than homosexual sex, blood transfusions, or drug use with infected needles.[3] This was an early step in understanding the differences between the African epidem-ic and what was going on back in North America. "Travel and frequent contact with prostitutes," Simonsen and Cameron suggested, "were associated with their seropositivity." They also noted that men who were uncircumcised were almost three times more likely to have an HIV infection, as were those who reported a history of genital ulcers. These were critical observations made very early on that, as the HIV/AIDS story unfolded, would come up persistently. "Uncircumcised men," the researchers noted, "were more frequently infected with HIV regardless of a history of genital ulcers. Our study finds that genital ulcers and an intact foreskin are associated with HIV infection in men with a sexually transmitted disease. Genital ulcers may increase men's susceptibility and they may increase the infectivity of women infected with HIV." The other upshot of this study was its progress toward defining and isolating "at-risk" groups, what Plummer was to call "the core group concept." An ongoing tension in Africa was between those who were trying to educate and target everybody and those who wanted to find out who the highest-risk groups were and concentrate on them.[4]

A study undertaken by Simonsen, Plummer, Ngugi, and a Canadian named Charleen Black with a cohort of 418 sex workers from lower socioeconomic strata (that is, shantytown women) made correlations between the 62 percent of these women who were HIV-positive and their Tanzanian origins.[5] This was also the research that identified the women's use of oral contraceptives as a possible factor in their HIV susceptibility. The findings were controversial, but the numbers were sobering. HIV rates of 60 percent among female sex workers who did not use oral contraceptives jumped to 80 percent among those who did.

All this study, research, and publishing necessitated—and created—a hive of activity. So rich was the territory of investigation and so urgent the need for more and new information that those on the ground felt compelled to take on as much research as could be financed by grant writing and could be handled by available personnel. Along with priorities, use of time and energies shifted. Frank Plummer, for example, estimated that from this time forward, up to half of his working hours were spent writing grant proposals, trying to get the support to undertake the research that pressed in from all sides.

Everything about the disease and the exploding epidemic that went with it was new, untested, puzzling, yet full of possibilities. The deadliness and speed of spread meant that those trying to understand the virus and contain it were pressed hard but likewise operated without a guidebook. To understand the African epidemic of HIV/AIDS demanded research, but research in exotic locales was in many ways a new business. In the West, careful protocols had been developed around medical research with human subjects, yet how did these hold in the furthest corners of Africa? On one level, the researchers might have felt like miners stumbling upon a rich vein on a far distant mountain, but could they just begin digging at will? What were the things to look out for, not just in the research itself, but in the protocols of how it was carried out? What were the cultural and political pitfalls that stood in the way? The Kenyans were at home, but the Canadians, Americans, Belgians, and British were not; they were guests in a place experiencing an urgent problem, but also a place whose cultural realities and assumptions differed dramatically from their own.

These questions are among the most sensitive in the rapidly expanding world of global health, and even early on a growing number of researchers realized they had much to struggle with. How could they be ethical, sensitive, and still effective? How could they avoid the worst designation put on their profession, that of "safari scientist," the hit-and-run artist who takes samples and then skedaddles, looking only to bolster personal research credentials. Michele Barry, a doctor in the Tropical Medicine and International Health Program at Yale University School of Medicine published an article in the *New England Journal of Medicine* in October 1988 that tried to grapple with the unique ethical considerations when undertaking scientific research with human subjects in "developing countries."[6] The article was clipped and photocopied broadly. The standard protocols, according to the Nuremberg Code and the Helsinki Declaration, Barry acknowledged, were Western, European, and North American. Faced now with an urgent situation in a different part of the world, what held? Researchers knew how to do things in the United States or Canada. Could you behave differently in Kenya?

A key issue in any research in the West was the autonomy of the participant and the matter of informed consent. In Africa, issues of "informed consent," suggested Barry, would possibly be interpreted differently. "Whereas in Western terms, selfhood emphasizes the individual," Barry wrote, "in certain African societies it cannot be extricated from a dynamic system of social relationships, both of kinship and of community as defined by the village. Thus an investigator seeking informed consent from persons in such a setting may need to approach community elders for their consent before attempting to obtain informed consent from individual persons. Clearly, the question of who gives informed consent—heads of households, elders, individual person, the tribe, the ministry of health, or the government—needs to be asked with cultural sensitivity."[7]

A significant factor centred around differing views of the balance between the individual and the community, or even the country. In the West, the primacy of the individual has become unassailable. "In non-autonomous populations," wrote Barry, "health policy decisions and risk-benefit analyses often place state interests above concern for the individual."[8] Individuals got sick and died, but the epidemic itself was a societal phenomenon affecting everything from a country's economy to its self-image in the world. Governments of African countries were torn between denial of AIDS and the urgency to learn more about what was causing and what might be done about this disease that in reality they could not deny. Barry cited an experience in Tanzania where government health officials insisted that, in a study to determine the prevalence of HIV infections among pregnant women, the women be told neither what they were being tested for nor the results. The rationale was that "the results could provoke hysteria within the population about a disease with no cure and for which limited resources were available, even for palliative treatment."[9]

Other things that needed to be dealt with by researchers attempting to operate in ethical fashion included illiteracy. How should they explain complicated investigations to persons who might have difficulty comprehending the explanations? Another was sensitivity to the capacities of the host countries. Many developing nations take pride, wrote Barry, in new scientific and laboratory achievements, and find it offensive when, for example, American investigators take African serum samples to the U.S. to be examined and processed. Tension around this raised its head periodically for the Canadians working in Nairobi, where they encountered apprehension and sometimes outright resistance when they wanted to carry samples back home. Another was the issue of publishing. The impulse of all scientists is to reach the most serious audience by getting published in the largest and most credible periodicals. In the world of medical research, no periodical supersedes the British *Lancet* or the American *New England Journal of Medicine*. If you have something to publish, those are the places you want to go first. What this meant, particularly in the early years when so much data was both urgent and astonishing, was that this data was frequently published internationally before it was shared with the host country. This was something that was further unsettling for Kenya. The Nairobi collaboration always included Kenyan researchers among the authors for its published papers, and these individuals knew of the data. But as has been noted in the previous chapter, there were occasions when the Kenyan government was surprised by data being published and was not pleased. The accompanying issue would have been how the government would have reacted had it been given a heads-up; had it then forbidden publication, what would the researchers have done? That would only serve to open new quandaries.

The program in Nairobi grew in terms of international participants; Peter Piot from the Institute of Tropical Medicine in Antwerp, Belgium, had been there since 1981. The University of Washington appeared on the scene in 1985. Financial support was international; during these years grants came via the Medical Research Council of Canada, IDRC, CIDA, the European Economic Community (EEC), the NIH, the American Foundation for AIDS Research, and the participating universities. By 1990, the joint project, Collaborative Research Centres, was able to boast substantial progress on a number of fronts. These included victories against genital ulcer disease and Haemophilus ducrey (the original issue to bring Ronald and Nsanze together), along with gonococcal infection and a whole plethora of sexually transmitted diseases. Working with new mothers and their babies at the Pumwani Maternal Hospital, Manitoban Robert Brunham and Belgian Marie Laga conducted trials to confirm that ophthalmic neonatorum, the bacterial infection contracted in the birth canal by babies whose mothers had gonorrhoea or chlamydia, which could lead to blindness, could be easily prevented with silver nitrate. This was a standard treatment in the developed world, but their work confirmed for the WHO that the treatment should become standard everywhere.[10] Sexually transmitted infections in mothers and their newborns became a target focussed on intensively by all the universities in the collaboration—Kenyan, Belgian, American, Canadian—leading to a long-term project as well as an important benchmark in HIV/AIDS science that would affect millions of future babies.

It is now known, decades later, that HIV can be transmitted across the placenta from mother to child before birth, and that infection also occurs at the time of delivery through exposure to an infected genital tract and, after birth, through breastfeeding. It is also known that the transmission of HIV is now preventable with antiretroviral drug treatment.[11] In the mid-1980s, all this was a vast unknown.

Twenty-five years on, Joanne Embree has come far in her career, occupying the chair of the medical microbiology department at the University of Manitoba. In August 1986, however, she was a young specialist in pediatrics and a post-doctoral fellow in infectious diseases preparing to head off to Kenya. The first HIV/AIDS cases there were, by then, a documented fact. The next idea, to pursue HIV research with pregnant women, came after researchers in Quebec found a fetus infected with HIV. It seemed imperative to undertake a similar search in Kenya. Plummer organized a team including Embree and Joan Kreiss, the University of Washington fellow who had just completed her studies with female commercial sex workers.

The project set up shop in the Pumwani Maternity Hospital and began to solicit a cohort of pregnant women. They secured an outpatient clinic, a room with space enough for a bed, a desk, a chair—though no sink. They found a translator and a nurse. The task, of course, was not only to gather samples, but also to have them tested. Serology was available in Kenya, but for quality assurance, Embree says they felt samples needed to be double-checked in First World labs. The concerns previously noted about the pride felt in developing countries about their new laboratory skills and their reluctance about exporting human samples notwithstanding, to act as the project did was deemed both prudent and necessary. So they went ahead. "Whoever among us was travelling would hand-carry the stuff," recalls Embree. "Peter Piot would carry a cooler to Antwerp, or Joan Kreiss would take one to Seattle or me to Canada." In some ways it seemed makeshift, but it was a heady time in research, the heyday of international cooperation. Everybody was in an adventurous spirit and prepared to muck in; too busy with exciting work for territorial disputes and turf wars to rear their heads.

Once the results started to come in from the mothers and babies, the researchers realized that, on this front too, there were going to be some groundbreaking conclusions. The transmission rate between pregnant mothers and newborn children was 20 percent. They were excited by the fact these numbers were a great deal lower than had been anticipated. "We set out thinking it would be more like 80 percent, and 50 percent of the babies would die within the first six months," says Embree. "We had even set that out as an estimate in our grant proposal." Mortality in their control group turned out to be 1 percent against the Kenyan national average of 10 percent, and the mortality of the babies from infected mothers was 10 percent, which equalled the rate in the general population. The reason for these pleasingly low rates, Embree concluded, were the same factors central to good maternal and newborn health across the world: good nutrition, anti-worming medicine so everybody had energy, up-to-date immunizations. "And if they came to us with infections, we made sure those were treated promptly and properly." In all too many places such standards continue to be elusive decades later. "All this had a huge impact," Embree recalls. "That's what I learned, good primary care makes all the difference."

All this time it had been difficult to publish their data. However, Kreiss undertook another controlled study and came up with remarkably similar numbers. Finally, the work was published in 1994 in the *Journal of Infectious Diseases*.[12] Their paper challenged conventional thinking. As Embree puts it, "If you have a good-news scientific study, it is easy to get published. If the news is not good—or differs significantly from conventional wisdom—you have to defend your work vigorously." In the long run their data prevailed. The CDC e-mailed Frank Plummer to tell him they'd looked at their database to find that corroborating data was there all along. Other institutions pulled out their databases and looked again at samples. Clearly, the Manitoba and Washington callaborators had done important primary work.

What they noted disturbingly, though, as they continued following their subjects, was that infants were acquiring HIV later on; children two years old were showing up newly infected with the virus. This development was puzzling. In response, Embree and Kreiss commenced testing every blood sample taken for HIV, even those of children who originally were negative. The tests started to pick up some mothers who had subsequently become HIV-positive—the result, they determined, of new exposures. But what had infected the children, especially those who had avoided infection at birth, despite having HIV-positive mothers?

"We were able," says Embree, "to see that a proportion of our kids were positive at birth, then negative at six months, but then became positive again." By this time, they had the means in Nairobi to do PCR (polymerized chain reaction), a testing tool that allowed them to see a virus. The team, including now a Kenyan researcher, Pratibha Datta, looked at their accumulating data and noted a pattern of transmission: 20 percent at one year was elevated to 44 percent after two years. "We were able," says Embree, "to plot out when infants became antibody negative. They would lose their antibodies between six and eighteen months of age, but because we kept testing we then found kids who were antibody positive. We found a two and a half year-old child who had been antibody positive, then negative, then positive again." When they looked at the family history, they realized what had happened: the mother had had another baby and, when breast-feeding her, had resumed breast-feeding the older child as well. This led to a logical conclusion: the children becoming HIV-positive had to be associated with continued breast-feeding. The researchers determined that the risk was cumulative; if a child was breast-fed by an infected mother beyond a year, the overall risk of transmission jumped to 44 percent.

To demonstrate this, Joan Kreiss, Ruth Nduati (later head of pediatrics at the University of Nairobi Medical School), and a young researcher from the University of Washington, Grace John-Stewart, set up a trial designed to be definitive. It was a randomized controlled trial, with one group of infants randomized to be breast-fed while another was formula-fed. The hypothesis was that if a mother was HIV-positive, she should formula-feed her child to reduce the risk of transmitting HIV. Randomized controlled trials are the gold standard of proof in medicine, and this one took several years to complete. But in the end, results corroborated the earlier observational findings: about half of HIV transmission from mother to child in a typical Kenyan population of HIV-positive mothers occurs because of breast-feeding.[13]

The fallout, of course, was that the information created an issue between breast-feeding advocates and those favouring formula feeding. Across the world, especially the developing world, the pressure to resist formula feeding was intense. The Swiss company, Nestlé, was under fire from those who championed the proven health—not to mention economic—value of breast-feeding for its aggressive marketing of baby formula. To have the HIV argument emerge on what many believed was the wrong side of this highly charged debate was dispiriting if not explosive and meant that there was a great deal of opposition from many quarters to conducting the trial. But it was an important new twist that could not be ignored, and in the end the researchers proved their point.[14] The information, however, also threw a wrinkle into Kenyan society. In traditional Kenyan culture, breast-feeding is not just one option among two; failing to do it is an immediate signal that something is wrong, and a stigma ensues. Family dynamics and relationships are disrupted, especially, as Embree points out, with a child named after parents or in-laws. It all raised very thorny problems for women; it was a touchy business for women not to breast-feed without revealing to families and neighbours the more difficult information of their HIV status. In response to this, the researchers knew they had to take on an active counselling role. "We counselled women," Embree says, "and encouraged them in diplomatic compromises, wean as soon as you can, reduce risk." It worked enough that consequently they saw the transmission rates go down.[15]

Canada's IRDC continued to finance the University of Manitoba Mother Child Health Clinic at the Pumwani Maternity Hospital. It was a busy hospital with a hundred new babies delivered each day. For their continuing study, the researchers selected part of that group, the Monday through Thursday deliveries. They encountered few refusals among the mothers, in part due to the Kenyan norm that it "would be impolite to say no." These mothers continued to provide researchers with their histories and agreed to show up at the clinic two weeks later. Most of them were as good as their word: the return rate was a substantial 80 percent. "We treated them well," recalls Embree. "Certainly in comparison to other city clinics. If you came to us, you'd get seen right away and treated for whatever ailed you."

Over the years, thousands of mothers joined the study, coming in droves right up until enrolment was stopped in 2000. By that point, studies in Uganda had shown that a single dose of the drug nevirapine during labour would reduce HIV transmission, and everything was changed. The Mother Child Health Clinic switched from being a research entity to a high-volume medical delivery and general clinic, looking after not only the mothers, but also fathers and siblings. Still later, by 2005, its operations moved to respond to the availability of funds from PEPFAR (the U.S. President's Emergency Plan For AIDS Relief) to provide antiretroviral therapies to patients with HIV/AIDS. The clinic, from that point on, would enrol patients who were HIV-positive and provide both antiretroviral drugs and counselling around the taking of the medication, which the patients would have to do for the rest of their lives. The mothers continue to serve as control groups for Plummer's studies on women who don't get HIV, comparing high-risk mothers who are also sex workers with the low-risk mothers (non-sex workers). The low-risk women are seen as an important comparison group, particularly if they come from the same ethnic group as the sex workers. Embree sums up by saying that "it was an exciting time. If we knew what we know now would we do it differently? Yes, but that's why we do research. Data that astounds you takes you on an entirely different research path."

Nothing anywhere in the project, however, came easily. A persistent bugbear was funding, getting sufficient money to do the work they believed needed doing. The home universities of the researchers like Plummer paid their salaries, but everything else from travel to support staff to equipment was found piece by piece by piece. They needed to make individual applications for individual grants. The overarching structures required to cover work that was growing rapidly in ambition and urgency simply weren't there. All support had to be negotiated at huge expenditures of energy and time; every win was a one-off and every need required a battle to fulfill it. In 1986 Plummer applied to the newly formed National AIDS Centre, part of the Canadian government's National Health Research and Development Program (NHRDP), for a grant to broaden research into heterosexual transmission of HIV and to identify risk patterns. He was turned down because the project for which he was requesting funds was not in Canada. He went ballistic. A letter fired off to the federal Minister of Health, Jake Epp (a prominent Manitoba representative in the Mulroney cabinet), began:

I am writing to you as a Canadian health researcher and a Manitoban to express my concern and frustration at Canadian funding for international health research, particularly regarding the acquired immunodeficiency syndrome (AIDS). This letter is prompted by the rejection of my proposal for a very important AIDS research project by the recently organized National AIDS Centre. The project proposal is enclosed for your information. Briefly, the project concerned the frequency and risk factors for heterosexual transmission of AIDS virus in Kenya. This issue is of concern to the world and can not be studied in Canada. The proposal was dismissed out of hand because the perceived venue was Kenya. Although I am challenging this decision through NHRDP, I think it is a symptom of deeper problems which I want to draw to your attention.

The deeper problems were that a parochial world lacked the mechanisms to adequately support what needed to be not domestic, but international research. The upshot of Plummer's letter-writing flurry was that his proposal was reconsidered and funding granted. But that was a single victory. Each attempt to get financing was a unique battle. In one twelve-month period, Plummer made eighteen grant proposals. His success rate was one in four.

Meanwhile, on the ground, things remained so ad hoc that, for the first years, Plummer didn't even have an office. There was the small lab space donated by the University of Nairobi, but the lead on-site scientist did most of his work from home. When he needed to meet anybody close to the university, the standard rendezvous spot was an outdoor table under a giant tree in the garden of the Hurlingham Hotel in an old English neighbourhood about a kilometre from Nairobi's university, or the window seat in a greasy restaurant called the Burger Chef across from the Barclays Bank in a little strip mall on Argwings Kodhek Road. Distracted by everything from passing traffic to noisy road construction, meetings were held and plans laid out, the participants fuelled by samosas, strong black coffee, and, in Plummer's case, Marlboro cigarettes. In 1988, the project finally did get a lab of its own, a modest building that came to be called "the Annex," on the grounds of the University of Nairobi Medical Faculty and adjacent to Kenyatta National Hospital. This was financed with $40,000 that Allan Ronald, now a kind of general fundraiser for the project, managed to secure from friends back in Winnipeg.[16] But bricks and mortar did not come to them automatically and, for the most part, the financial continuation of the project itself was never something that could be taken for granted.

Things were not a great deal better for anyone else. The University of Washington, with funding from the NIH, had the largest STD research program in the world. The money had allowed them, since 1972, to provide fellowships to pre- and post-doctoral students to work either domestically or internationally. In the late 1980s these Fogarty AIDS International Training and Research Program (AITRP) grants provided $1 million a year. As a result, the University of Washington became a magnet for people who wanted to work abroad in the field of STD research. After King Holmes connected with Kenya via the Nairobi collaboration in the mid-1980s, more than eighty Kenyans, including the collaboration's key participants such as Joshua Kimani, Kawango Agot, and J.O. Ndinya-Achola, came to the U.S. to study at the University of Washington. In turn, at least twenty-five UW students travelled to Kenya. Thus, on one level, that American university operated under a better funding situation than the Canadians. But they had no better luck than the Canadians in providing an overarching umbrella to give structural security to their foreign enterprises. In fact, the buildings the Americans worked out of in Nairobi were constructed with Canadian dollars.[17]

The Canadians got financing in later years, again with Ronald and to some degree Plummer cobbling it together, for two more lab and office buildings, each a bigger replacement for the one before it. One, built in 1996, was financed by the government of Canada through the High Commission in Kenya. Then, in 2007, came the crowning legacy of Plummer's almost two-decade career in Kenya, a well-appointed new laboratory complete with Level 3 biotech security and funded overwhelmingly by the Canada Foundation for Innovation. The Canadians as well, in 1990, finally scored with CIDA to finance the long-hoped for country-wide project to strengthen STD/HIV control in Kenya (as described in Chapter 3). They signed a contract for five years at $1 million per year, the most significant money they'd had up until that point.

Every system with which they operated over the years had to be invented, often from scratch. A case in point was the shipping of supplies halfway around the world from North America to East Africa. Leslie Slaney began her career at the University of Manitoba in 1978, just in time to help arrange supply and support for Margaret Fast, the first of the Manitobans to set up residence in Nairobi. The strategy, for Fast, was to have her take most of her own supplies with her. What she didn't carry, or what it emerged she needed as the year progressed, was mailed to her through the post. The substantial downside to the mail service, admits Slaney, was the risk that items might disappear at the other end. An alternate system, set up by Frank Plummer, was to send items to an American embassy contact in New York, from whence, piggybacking on a system the American Centers for Disease Control already had set up, they would be sent on to Nairobi through a US Army delivery. However, the most reliable and most used method, was for project personnel travelling to Nairobi to carry things with them—any number of items large and small—load them onto the plane on which they were flying, and, if need be, shell out for excess baggage charges.

As the work expanded and demand increased for supplies, some of them large items of scientific equipment like centrifuges and refrigerators, the travelling scientists could no longer be expected to carry these in excess baggage. The solution was to start making shipments by boat. The first sea shipment from Canada to Nairobi was sent to supply the new Annex lab in 1990. A sea shipment meant that supplies were collected in Winnipeg, transported by rail to Halifax, loaded onto a ship that then travelled across the Atlantic, through the Mediterranean and the Suez Canal, and on to Kenya's Indian Ocean port of Mombasa. Alternately, it went down the Atlantic coast of Africa and, after rounding the Cape of Good Hope, eventually docked at Mombasa. For his part, Ian Maclean frequently tried to be in Kenya at the time of a shipment's arrival in order to facilitate the completion of the journey and make sure everything arrived in good shape. He would travel with his personal tool kit of wrecking bar and hammers to take the crates apart and free the enclosed cargo. One of the most colourful and exciting moments was when the goods at last rolled up to the Nairobi lab on the back of a lorry from the customs depot. Unloading and uncrating was a big job requiring many hands. There was, to begin with, no forklift available in Nairobi so the crates had to be shunted from the truckbed manually. This was achieved by circling them with ropes and sliding them down planks, an exceedingly labour-intensive undertaking. Maclean made sure enough hands were available by promising that anybody who helped could then make a claim on the plywood and materials that had crated the shipment. Wood being in ever short supply for many people in Kenya meant that good three-quarter-inch plywood was coveted because it could be taken home and transformed into shelves, tables, an outbuilding, almost anything. Nothing was wasted. Not only the plywood was in demand, but so were the two-by-fours that framed the crates. Even the nails were pulled and straightened for re-use. The unloading turned into a festive afternoon that brought out everybody, from lab workers to project drivers and, on at least one occasion, Dr Omu Anzala, who would one day become chair of the medical microbiology department but on this day, with his sleeves fully rolled up, helped make short and happy work of a big job.

The shipping of materials and supplies from North America to Kenya was one thing, but important cargo came in the other direction too. This was the plasma, serum, and human tissue specimens that the researchers had collected for study—some of it analyzed in Kenya, but much of it wanting further study in labs back home. It is easy to forget how recent are the innovations that actually make all such specimen shipment possible. In 1927, Fritz Trenz, a Swiss doctor and missionary working in Gabon, West Africa, faced the puzzle of how to transport vibrio cholera bacteria to his laboratory at home in Strasbourg, France. He reached the conclusion he had no alternative but to drink a vial containing the bacteria. He knew what would happen but gulped it down anyway. On board ship he predictably became deathly ill with fever and other dastardly side effects, but once back in France was able to extract a healthy specimen— from his own body. With freezing, refrigeration, and air transportation, transfer of specimens has come a long way since Fritz Trenz.

Originally, in the spirit of each researcher with his or her overweight luggage, many travelling back to Canada or the United States or Belgium had coolers (the kind you might take on a picnic) in which they carried frozen specimens. They checked these with their luggage and hoped there would be no problems. At their destination, the researchers might have to explain the contents to customs, but the only officials ever remotely interested were from the ministries of agriculture, concerned about animal diseases. About human diseases, nobody batted an eye.

In Kenya protocols around export permits were developed, but not without moments of friction and sometimes mistrust between the foreigners and their Kenyan hosts. The matter of foreign scientists taking samples out of the country was not one all Kenyans, even the project's collaborators within the University of Nairobi, were consistently comfortable with (see chapter three). During the years when Isaac Wamola was chair of the microbiology department (1987-90) there were some tense moments around this practice.

Eventually such matters were sorted out and specimen shipment in larger quantities ensued. New technologies for doing this shipping had also become available. For a while, the method of choice was liquid nitrogen tanks. Thirty litres of liquid nitrogen surrounding specimens would keep them frozen. The problem was that things could spill if the tanks fell over, and occasionally they did. Such an occurrence would result in a middle-of-the-night call to Ian Maclean or Kelly MacDonald from the British Airways warehouse at Pearson Airport in Toronto and, occasionally, lost material. After 2000, another technical change allowed the project to use dry shippers, which entailed a liquid nitrogen tank whose walls were lined with foam. These were expensive, $4,000 each, with shipping costs of $1,000 each way. One instance of sending live HIV to or from Nairobi would cost $3,500 including permits.

Over the decades, equipment became increasingly expensive, both laboratory equipment and, something that came on the scene at about the same time as the project got started in the early 1980s, computers. Loe Dierick, husband of the Belgian pediatrics researcher Marleen Temmerman, living in Nairobi with his wife and son, offered to help Plummer get the project computerized. In 1986 he set up a first version PC-AT with an Intel 80286 processor and a 10 MB hard drive. "It was a big machine," Dierick recalls, "that would get so warm it attracted geckoes who laid their eggs in it." A year later, in 1987, the PC-AT was replaced by three 286s loaded with a database program called VA Fileman, named after the veterans' administration that had pioneered its use. By 1990, well ahead of the days of easy e-mail, Dierick played around with modems from U.S. Robotics to get data back to Canada. Plummer was a keen computer user, recognizing the potential for both data processing and communication that the emerging technology promised.

But all of this cost money. A young doctor from Nova Scotia, Neil Simonsen, was Plummer's graduate fellow at the time. The frustration, as he recounts it, was that information on HIV/AIDS in Africa was becoming known, but it took time—as long as a decade or more—for donors to redirect money. Meanwhile, they needed lots of it; they had teams of people to pay if they were going to do things right, and they had equipment to purchase. Plummer tended to go out and buy whatever he felt he needed and ask permission later. Repeatedly, this landed him in trouble with his administrator back home in the offices of the medical microbiology department in Winnipeg. Things rarely happened without drama. Plummer was either seen as behind the game in the matter of his payments, or ahead of it in his perception of needs. Ian Maclean explains that "he would recognize the need for something, computers or a piece of equipment that would cost $75,000, and he would just buy it." When this happened, the administrators back in Winnipeg would have to scramble. For many years, the job of scrambling fell to Theresa Birkholz, who started working for the University of Manitoba in 1964 and, until she retired in 2000, was in charge of operating budgets and grants for the department of medical microbiology.

"Frank could never stay in budget," she complains. "He was always buying lab equipment or project vehicles." If the grants didn't specify such items by name, or if the purchases exhausted the budget, she would be forced to write letters to funding agencies and "beg for 10% leeway." She did this regularly but, eventually, to make things work and insure against surprises or catastrophe, she developed some tricks of her own. She got into the habit of holding back part of each grant so that when the inevitable crisis came along, she would be able to reach into a drawer and produce a surprise $40,000. "If the grant was $200,000 I saved $40,000 so that when the crunch came, we'd be able to manage. I didn't tell Frank the whole story, it was my form of protection."

Yet scientifically, Plummer would turn out to be right and doing what he did, according to people like Ian Maclean, "kept us ahead of the game." Maclean offers a whole list of technologies that, through the years, Plummer's intuition, as much as anything else, told him he needed to get hold of, pronto. These included numerous diagnostic and research technologies that were developed between 1980 and 2000. PCR (polymerase chain reaction) is a diagnostic tool to amplify DNA. Getting access to it helped researchers at the Pumwani Maternity Hospital identify HIV in their babies. Early on, the researchers were able to test for HIV by antibodies. With PCR, they no longer needed antibodies; they could now look for the virus using new diagnostic tools to identify infected people. "Frank was good at making sure we had the latest equipment," says Maclean. "Theresa will tell you she was pulling her hair out. But in many cases technology was moving too fast. A new thermal-cycler that they would use to do the amplification of the DNA from the HIV could cost $15,000 which had not been budgeted for, but he needed it tomorrow so he'd go and spend the money." Computers were another item that they realized would be useful very early on, in the early 1980s. "Before anybody at the University of Manitoba had a computer," according to Maclean, "Frank had to have one in Nairobi. But it paid off. We had this massive amount of data and Nico (Nagelkerke) came in and with his Kaplan-Meier plot was able to set up models that led to the discovery of the resistant women. Frank is one of these guys, 'we need it, who cares.' And in the end he was proven right."

There were also frustrations with the research. With this new disease right smack in front of them, there was a lot to do. But the landscape was wide open; what directions should the quest go in? The logical research paths were those that figured out how to minimize the spread of the epidemic, but which of those, like oral contraception, would erupt into controversy? King Holmes told Plummer to expect frustrations. "There are three stages surrounding the acceptance of new research," he told him. "First, people will say it's not true. Second, they will say it's true but it's not important. Third they will say it's true and we knew it all along." In other words, heading off to find hypotheses, especially if they were novel or counterintuitive, was an often thankless task.

A case in point was a decision to pursue what they had been looking at in Nairobi for half a decade already, other sexually transmitted infections. The novel twist would be to determine if or how HIV risk might be connected. Were more "traditional" sexually transmitted diseases, particularly ones with lesions and open sores, potential conduits for the new infection? Plummer put Simonsen and another young trainee, Bill Cameron, in charge of an investigation that culminated in a paper published in 1988 in the *New England Journal of Medicine*, showing that among men with sexually transmitted infections, HIV infections were higher than among their peers.[18]

But this once more raised people's skeptical antennae. The WHO in Geneva responded by convening an expert group to discuss the relationship between STIs and HIV and summoned Plummer. He was apprehensive, believing that the meeting was "basically set up to discredit our data." Peter Piot, his former collaborating colleague in Nairobi, still some years away from taking over responsibility for AIDS for the United Nations, chaired the meeting, and later confirmed Plummer's suspicions. Before Plummer even arrived, a communiqué had been drafted to explain that there was no proven relationship between HIV and other STDs. However, things went off the rails. Before Plummer spoke, two presenters laid out how in epidemiological studies one needed to prove causation. The accepted way to do this was to apply something called the Bradford-Hill criteria. Professor Thierry Mertens, who worked for WHO, gave a presentation on Bradford-Hill. But Plummer was prepared to counter: "It so happened," he says, "that my presentation was set up against these criteria and most everything was met." A second presenter was completing a study in which she was finding no relationship between STIs and HIV. The problem, soon pointed out, was that she had few STIs in her study group. In the end, Plummer carried the day, the tide turned, and congratulations were offered all round. "They had to rewrite the communiqué," Plummer reported with satisfaction. "It was still difficult for much of the world to accept the reality of heterosexual transmission of HIV," is how Piot explains it. "Gays owned AIDS as their disease. But that the virus would respect gender barriers didn't make sense. We argued that; we were the pioneers."

CHAPTER FIVE

Secrets of the Sex Workers

I n January 2010 I went to the Majengo clinic to meet a woman named Hawa Chelangat. In the heat of mid-morning I walked from my hotel to Kenyatta Hospital and the Nairobi collaboration's brand new laboratory and office building, then caught a ride across town in the standard manner, Mr D's van. When we arrived at the shantytown clinic, nurse Jane Kamene was there to greet us with Hawa in tow. This was a reunion rather than a first meeting, and when Hawa and I saw each other, we were both all smiles. It was thirteen years since we had first known each other, and how time had flown. Back then she was thirty-seven and living with her four children, all young and in school. Now she had turned fifty, her children were grown, and she had a grandchild. Only her daughter, Asha, mother of the grandchild, still lived in the shantytown. But Hawa looked good. She remained petite, with flawless smooth skin and shining eyes, and was well dressed, as I'd remembered her, in a colourful Muslim hijab. She'd also just gotten married, she told us, Jane translating to cover the great gap between Hawa's halting English and my meagre Swahili, and appeared delighted by this new status as wife of a man named Abdul. Not much else had changed, however. She still lived in her hut at the far end of the shantytown, close to the community water tap and a ten-minute walk from the clinic. She still made her living from sex and still had her clients who she met in her front room, presumably when Abdul was away. She still came to the clinic where Jane Kamene and the doctors took samples of her blood regularly and kept an eye on her health. And, yes, she was still HIV-negative.

This HIV status for Hawa was the important thing, the reason for my having wanted to make a film about her back in 1997; the reason for the continued interest researchers at the clinic had in her. And this negative status remained the evidence

68

that she carried something within her, in the makeup of her body or her genetic structure, that might yet be unlocked to help solve the great puzzle of HIV/AIDS.

Our film about Frank Plummer's research had been made for the National Film Board of Canada and had been called *Searching for Hawa's Secret*. The title, we believed, said it all. By 1977 Plummer's research had taken a dramatic turn and Hawa, the shantytown sex worker supporting her four children, was a critical piece. Four years before that, in the summer of 1993, he had flown to Berlin, the newly constituted capital of the newly unified Germany, for the ninth International AIDS Conference. These meetings had started in 1985 as annual affairs drawing medical researchers together to exchange information and give one another courage against the challenges they faced with the burgeoning disease. A decade later, they had grown exponentially into almost iconic gatherings of what had become (and would continue to grow into) an "AIDS establishment." AIDS, unlike any other disease, had taken on a worldwide aura. It was still uncurable, looking ever more like an unsolvable medical mystery that could hardly even be contained. Yet—maybe because of this, plus the deaths of high-profile victims like the actor Rock Hudson—it garnered the horrified fascination of all kinds of people, including Hollywood celebrities like Elizabeth Taylor, and meeting about AIDS attracted not just medical people and scientists, but also activists, politicians, anybody with a point to make. After 1996, the meetings were convened every two years, rather than annually, with the additional gap only making them bigger and more substantial: they started to press into the territory of the World's Fair, or even the Olympics. As if to additionally focus their direction, the meetings started to be given theme labels. The 1989 gathering in Montreal had been "The Scientific and Social Challenges of AIDS"; 1990 in San Francisco was "AIDS in the Nineties, From Science to Policy." As the decades turned, the thematic language became more urgent, reflecting the expanding political, cultural, and legal interests that accompanied the natural interest of medical science. For Mexico City in 2008, the theme was a battle cry: "Universal Action Now." The meeting in the summer of 2010 in Vienna was titled "Rights Here, Rights Now."

The Berlin conference in 1993 had no stated thematic title, but for Frank Plummer it might have been labelled his coming out. Plummer had been to these events before, even causing a stir in 1987 with his revelation about a connection between oral contraceptives and HIV. In Berlin he would make a stir again. The world was fascinated by AIDS. Journalists attended the international meetings in ever greater numbers and covered them with ever-growing intensity, looking for headlines to satisfy the hungry and, to a large degree, frightened global public: what, they wanted to know and report back, was the latest news on the scientific front? What were the latest casualty numbers? Why wasn't there as yet a cure or even a vaccine? As the conference in Berlin progressed, a well-placed and knowledgeable journalist stalking the event was Jon Cohen, a writer for the Washington-based *Science* magazine. In its pre-event issue, Cohen had produced an article alerting conference participants about sessions not to be missed. One of these, he said, was a session that would be addressed by a Canadian working in Kenya who had come upon an enticing new wrinkle. When Plummer got to the appointed hall, he found it already crowded with those who had heeded Jon Cohen's directions. It was an expectant lot, and he didn't disappoint. What he had found, he announced, was not a cure or a vaccine, but something almost equally fascinating. Having followed his group of Pumwani-Majengo sex workers by then for almost ten years, he had seen many get sick and die. But his news was that he had detected a small subset within them—some twenty-four women, about 5 percent of the total enrolment—who, despite being exposed repeatedly to HIV and only infrequently using protective measures like condoms, never became infected with the virus. Their friends and co-workers were infected, becoming sick and dying, but this small group were not. Plummer and his colleagues, who would get their paper on the discovery published in the *Lancet* in 1996, had determined that they had encountered a resistance, maybe even an immunity.[1]

Lots of attention was lavished on Plummer in Berlin, but when he got back to Nairobi in October the deluge truly landed. A freelance journalist from the U.K. named Elizabeth Jones arrived in Nairobi primed to produce articles for the *Guardian* newspaper and documentary pieces for both BBC television and radio. As the stories made their way out and other media caught on, one thing led to another. Canal+ arrived from France; Canadian media called. "It was absolute pandemonium," Plummer's associate, Neil Simonsen, recalls. "One day there were seventeen interviews." The researchers believed they were on to something very big, and the world agreed.

"There's nothing," Frank Plummer told me one afternoon, "quite like the rush you get when you discover something new. It's better than any drug you could ever imagine." We were sitting in the small office he kept in the house he and his family occupied on a pleasant, heavily shaded road that dead-ended at a coffee plantation. He was animated to the point of agitation, his eyes shining with unsuppressed excitement, his hands alternately fiddling with a ballpoint pen and then tapping the keys of his computer keyboard. By that spring, in 1997, he had discovered the beginning of an intricate chain of commonality among what were by then being called his cadre of resistant sex workers. His thoughts turned to the legendary stories about how Edward Jenner, the country doctor in Berkeley, had come upon the milkmaids who did not fall ill with smallpox when one of the frequent epidemics raged through eighteenth-century England. It occurred to Jenner that because of the job the young women did they'd been exposed to cowpox and that was the factor that made them resistant to the much worse disease. That discovery provided one of the first insights into the human immune system and permitted a vaccine to be developed to protect from smallpox. How had Jenner felt, Plummer caught himself wondering, when he had come to that understanding? How long had it taken to realize the full ramifications of his finding?

Plummer's imagination wanted him to be on the edge of something that might turn out to have equivalent world-shaking import. The continent of Africa was overrun with theories about HIV/AIDS, some of them voodoo-like and bizarre. That very week, the local Nairobi newspaper, the *Nation*, carried separate reports that the disease was not a virus, that it was a Western plot, and that it could be cured by honey. Likewise, Africa had been taken over by a plethora of bona fide AIDS researchers looking at everything from the nature of the disease to the nature of its spread to the potential for vaccines. On top of that there was a growing number of researchers looking into social and economic impacts. Among all these, Plummer and his associates knew their project was only one brick in the vast wall. But because of the information that had come to them and its surprising nature, they had been able to turn a dramatic corner.

Science is the methodical verification of answers to questions that are posed as hypotheses. It happens with the gathering of data through the endless taking of samples and reducing them to cogent bits of information, and then a similarly endless poring over that information. It is a combination of detective work plus statistics plus the application of theories or models of predictability and probability. Thanks to technologies such as computers, material that would have taken months or years to sort and calculate in the past can now be tabulated in seconds. But what is still required is the human mind to make the choice to say, let's go down *this* pathway rather than some other one, let us ask *this* question among all possible questions. Plummer had all kinds of numbers and statistics garnered from the blood work done with the sex workers. Day after day technicians peered down their microscopes, entering whatever information they found into the bank of data. Then, usually at night, the scientist would sit in the dark of his home study, only illuminated by the glow of the computer screen, worrying over the results, trying to trace patterns, looking for anomalies.

He would have had a difficult time reaching his conclusions without the help of his team, in particular his chief number cruncher, a rumpled statistician from Holland named Nico Nagelkerke. Nagelkerke was already in Nairobi, doing work for KEMRI, when Plummer was directed to him. Plummer considered him brilliant. Through their day-by-day testing of the women, Plummer's researchers had amassed a huge amount of information. But what had to happen then, as one of the associates put it, "was Nico messing around with his statistical modelling and Kaplan-Meier Plot, following trends and in this case, finding that the curve went down and then levelled off. If everybody had equal chance of dying the curve would eventually go to zero. But in this case it did not, it levelled off."[2]

Plummer's eureka moment, coming one night while he was sitting alone, poring over his screen, was the realization that he should focus his questing attention not on the women who were infected but those, like Hawa, who remained infection-free. If they could figure out for certain what it was that was keeping these women out of harm's way, they might be onto something huge. In short order, he came to the conclusion that the information he had was good enough for him to suspect an actual immunity, a natural immunity that was peculiar to these women. His next thought was this: would it be possible to extract that and bottle it and thereby protect everybody? Long-time associate Ian Maclean described both Plummer and the process again: "The classic Frank is the thinker. He would sit up in his office all night and just look at data with his brain going 'ca-ching, ca-ching'. Then he gets the rest of us to implement his ideas."

Hawa had been part of the project from almost the beginning. When my crew and I showed up ready to make our film in early 1997, she had been involved since 1986, more than ten years, faithfully, at least once a week making her appearance in order to keep her end of the bargain with the researchers. Her project number was 935, which meant that a lot of women had been enrolled before her, but a good many had been enrolled after as well. She came to us through a kind of lottery. By now, three years post-Berlin, the number of women who were labelled, carefully, "persistent sero-negatives," had climbed to sixty women.

The definition could be applied to any woman who had been active as a sex worker for at least three years yet remained uninfected by HIV. Because of all the attention, ours was not the first film crew to arrive, and demand for women to participate in everything from interviews to short news items to full-blown films had been brisk. The clinic responded by trying to impose some sense of order. It instituted two things: those media representatives demanding time from the women would have to pay them for their lost earnings—plus a little extra; and the women would be given turns to participate in interviews or productions—determined through the lottery. This is how Hawa ended spending the next weeks with us and we with her.

The harsh truth is that, sympathetic as we might be, it is almost impossible for anyone from the "comfortable" side of the world to properly comprehend the life of someone who lives in a tin-roofed shack in a shantytown and sells sex for a living. The clash of sensibilities is inevitable; the very sounds and smells and crowding of personal space for the outsider is not so much offensive as frightening. At best it is intriguing. Then there is grappling with the idea of laying oneself down several times a day, disrobing or partially disrobing, going through a sex act, pulling oneself back together, accepting some money, saying goodbye to the customer, and getting ready to do it all over again. Our impetus is to judge or feel sympathy either for the person or the circumstances, but to come to an actual understanding is an almost impossible reach. For starters, though selling sex is not an occupation of high social standing in the shantytowns of Nairobi, neither is it looked on with the same pejorative disdain—or for that matter pity—as it is looked upon in the West. Sex in one way is easier, it is something most everybody does; if you want to sell or buy it, so be it. This is not to say there isn't a power imbalance between someone for whom that is the only option and the rest of the community, but there is not the hand-wringing approbation with which both sellers and buyers get looked upon in most of the West. At the same time, life is hard—as it is hard for everybody in these shantytowns, whether they are selling sex or pineapples. Theirs is a hand-to-mouth existence. Money is scarce, saving any is a near impossibility, a day off sick— or a sick child—is a disaster. When your hut is built from scraps of plywood, sheet metal, cardboard, and mud, and the street running in front of your door is packed mud with an open ditch down the middle to handle sewage, the rainy season as well is a disaster. Yet life prevails. People laugh, they love, they procreate, they raise their children, they do their laundry, they cook their suppers, they congregate. You would have to look far to find rooms as tidy and well swept as the little chambers of the sex workers. Lace doilies adorn chairs dragged in from the rubbish heap or tables made from cast-off crating; the walls are decorated with cheery pictures cut from magazines and calendars.

Nonetheless, these women were the ones faced with a devastating new disease they'd never before heard of; a work-related illness they could catch from their customers or pass on to their customers, a deadly disease that if they got pregnant they could pass on to their new baby. And now they were approached by professional-looking people in white lab coats. Some of them were white foreigners, others young Kenyan doctors and nurses, and all were telling the women they had a role to play in understanding, maybe even curing, the disease. It was a lot to expect by the foreigners and a lot to take in for the women. But they took it on, an addition to their lives that must have seemed like an extra job, for the most part an unpaid job, save in the abstract of potentially saving their lives or those of their children and grandchildren.

It was through making the film that I was able to get a window into the insistent dedication of both the women enrolled in the project and the staff in the steady, tedious task of trying to glean cellular information that some expert might be able to do something with. Once in the clinic, with our camera rolling, Hawa showed us how it worked. She went through the same sequence of procedures as the women ahead of her in line, which all of them had been doing for years. The presiding clinician in those days was a precise, scholarly young man, Ephantus Njagi, and the clinical nurse, a calm, motherly woman named Joann Ambani. As our camera operator pointed his lens, Njagi straightened the collar on his white jacket and nurse Joann stepped closer in a hovering manner to be ready to provide translation. It all took a while. Though the day we were there was a hot one, Hawa was in layers of clothing; beneath her robe she had a dark blue sweatshirt, under that a t-shirt. Finally she was able to stick out a bare arm into which Njagi stuck the first of several needles. As the blood pulsed into the vials, Joann affixed a label to each: "patient number 935." "Because she is sero-negative," she explained, "we need more from her. We watch her even more closely than the others." Everyone was careful not to make too many open assumptions, but had, at any time, her tests come back positive instead of negative, it would have been devastating, and not just to her personally.

Each vial of blood from each of the women was plugged with a colour-coded top: red, purple, green, yellow, to designate its destination once back downtown in the lab. All samples would first be tested for HIV using a test called "ELISA." From there they would then enter a vast system of research corridors to break them down into every conceivable component part: the blood would be peered at under microscopes, spun in centrifuges, frozen in liquid nitrogen, transported thousands of miles by air to Toronto and Winnipeg. The cells would be examined a multitude of different ways, all in the hope of yielding information, not just about the person from whom it had been taken, but more global information about the immune system of the human race and the diabolical virus that was attacking it. As the morning wore on, the crowd in the waiting room grew. The sheer numbers of people waiting in queue made it seem like the process at the clinic might never end, yet, miraculously, shortly after noon everybody had been attended to. The staff tidied up, locked the doors, and, carrying their coolers filled with the morning's collected specimens, piled back into Mr D's van for the return trip to the university and the labs.

Plummer, by this time, had a small army of colleagues, associates, and staff. These included not only researchers from Winnipeg and Nairobi, but also from Seattle and Oxford. One of the Canadians, Keith Fowke, had made his first visit to Nairobi in 1990 as Plummer's graduate student ready to spend three months with the sex workers at the clinic. The research strategy was to use radioactive T cell assays, and Fowke recalls hauling lead-lined shields to Kenya because there were no radiology labs in Nairobi and he had to bring everything from Canada. "The shields were really heavy," he recalls. Yet being able to import them so easily was a luxury: "You wouldn't get away with hauling lead-lined shields through airport security these days," he notes. Fowke was young and saw everything as an adventure, even the necessity of living and working under less than the best conditions. The challenge of the work provided the payoff. "The first piece of data we got that suggested that these women were exposed to HIV but not infected came from this radioactive T cell assay," he recounts. "I took the printout and then had to go home and work out the math and figure out the background and how much of the cell killing was specific to HIV infected cells. I was sitting in the apartment having a cold Tusker beer while doing all my math and realizing about the cells I was looking at, 'Wow, they're not fighting an HIV infection and it looks real.' It was an ecstatic moment; it was not a theory anymore, we had some data that suggested this was really happening. I remember calling Frank, telling him about it and being really happy."

Along with Fowke were other young scientists who first encountered the project as students, and for whom, without doubt, trips to Africa were coveted perks. One of these was Kelly MacDonald. While happy to work in the lab back in Canada, MacDonald found that forays into the front-line clinics helped her both gain and keep perspective, giving grounding to the theoretical and making everything not abstract but real, not to mention more poignant. "This is easy on a theoretical basis, when you're looking at molecules," she observed one afternoon after a session in the clinic. "But when you encounter people directly and see their faces, when they're laughing and joking with you, when you give them the pills for their pneumonia and understand that the six kids sitting outside are all their children, then it's harder." She paused for a moment, her eyes misting over, then went on: "Sometimes I retreat behind the science because otherwise it's just too overwhelming. I really like these people." Time in the field had helped the young researcher who would eventually head up an HIV vaccine project at Toronto's Mount Sinai Hospital understand something else about her profession: "You can't cure all these people," she said, "so you go back to your lab and do the research because maybe that's the way you can do some good."

Numerous contacts and relationships developed through pure word of mouth. Rupert Kaul was a young medical student specializing in infectious diseases at the University of Toronto in 1994 when Kelly MacDonald, just arrived in Toronto from Manitoba, suggested he might talk to Frank Plummer if he wanted some interesting research and clinical experience. MacDonald helped Kaul get in touch with Plummer, whom he then arranged to meet at an upcoming conference in Bethesda, Maryland. Kaul was curious how, at a conference with thousands of people, he was going to recognize Plummer. "Keep an eye out for Grizzly Adams," MacDonald told him.

Kaul and Plummer hit it off, and Kaul soon found himself working closely with his new mentor. Plummer invited him to Nairobi, telling him he would be able to engage in some work around immune responses and HIV. "You can go to the clinic and enroll people, we'll have a technician on the site to run the assays, you can put together the database," Kaul recalls Plummer telling him. The University of Toronto arranged a year's worth of funding and off he went. Optimism notwithstanding, things don't always go as we wish them to, and Kaul's year turned into a frustrating one, starting with the flat he had been given to stay in getting burglarized the first night he was there.[3] The promised research technician didn't materialize, something he says Plummer tried to rectify by bringing out a lab technician named John Rutherford from Manitoba to teach Kaul technical skills. It was one step forward and two back as more frustrations got added to the list: he discovered that certain assays didn't work, then he learned from

Keith Fowke that some of the antibodies they depended on were in a freezer that had broken down several times. "It was all very discouraging," admitted Kaul. "By the time the year ended I'd done one little clinical epidemiology project and none of the immunology research had worked. But I was working at the clinic with patients and that was satisfying." His funding, however, had finished, so Kaul found himself having to choose whether to go back home "with my tail between my legs not having accomplished much," or find a way to stay longer. The satisfactions of the clinical work were enough to persuade him to try to stay on.

It was one thing to come to the conclusion that a certain number of sex workers in a fetid Nairobi slum might be immune to HIV. But the critical question, in fact the only useful question, remained: why? What protection did Hawa and the others in the small group of women have that nobody else had? This, then, became the task for the scientists, to set up a whole new set of questions and hypotheses to help them travel usefully through that quest, searching, isolating, testing. By 1997, and the time we were making our film, Plummer's researchers had identified at least one commonality among the resistant women: they all shared similar HLA. Human leukocyte antigens, for the uninitiated, are cell markers that everybody possesses. But the significant thing is that not everybody has the same ones nor do we have them in the same combinations; there are a variety of types and they come in a variety of combinations. As the HLA taken from the white blood cells in the serum samples of the sex workers was typed in the lab and the information put into a database, what had become apparent was that the resistant women had rare types of HLA and that the combinations of HLA molecules in the resistant women took on similar patterns. If one wanted to look for the characteristics that separated these women from all the others, this, the scientists believed, was important. They knew that the job of the HLA molecule, perched on the surface of every human cell, was to function as a sort of traffic light, telling visitors when to proceed or when to stop. When it saw the approach of cells it didn't like, for example, it would summon surveillance cells to destroy them. That, in a nutshell, is how the immune system works. So if the HLA combinations peculiar to the resistant women were what was turning on the red light to halt the entry of the HIV virus, then that could be considered important.

The HLA line of inquiry was important for another reason. It meant that the resistant women were being protected by something that was cellular in nature rather than triggered by antibodies. One way the body's immune system works is that when a foreign virus invades, antibodies are created. Most vaccines, in fact, pursue this line of defense; a tiny bit of virus is introduced into the body in order to activate antibodies which will then do their work, like cruising police cars targeting any future arrival of recognizable foreign cells. The smallpox vaccine works like this, and it was how the cowpox antibodies were able to fight the smallpox virus in the milkmaids. But HIV is different. No vaccine producer as yet believes they can afford to introduce even the tiniest bit of that virus into a human body. It is too dangerous and too volatile; once introduced it could not be controlled and the outcome could not be predicted. However, were one able to depend on the cellular response of HLA, rather than the production of antibodies, that could all be avoided. A vaccine based on HLA would fight HIV without the dangerous tactic of introducing any of the virus itself into the body.

An additional twist, though, soon offered itself. One of the Kenyan doctors, Joshua Kimani, a young protege of Plummer's who had studied in Seattle and Winnipeg, taking full advantage of the collaboration after getting his medical degree in Nairobi, pointed out that a number of the uninfected women were related to one another. Kimani understood Africa's intricate kinship webs, and recognized that of the women, some were sisters or half-sisters, others were cousins—first cousins and distant cousins—and from the same parts of rural Kenya. He explained this to Plummer, who decided immediately to follow it up scientifically. Was it just coincidental that some of the women were related to one another, or might the HLA patterning and the resistance itself be genetic? Was it something families shared and, that, therefore, could be inherited? He decided to pursue it by asking a number of the women, including Hawa, to help the researchers track down their relatives.

Hawa came from a region in the western part of Kenya, in the tea country in the direction of Lake Victoria. Her parents were dead, but her extended family all lived back there. The researchers prepared to pay a visit to these brothers and sisters and cousins and gather as much information as possible from them. A host of tasks would be part of such a visit: blood samples would have to be taken and brought back to determine the HLA types; everybody would need to be tested for HIV. Plummer held a meeting to plot out a strategy. He himself was not going to lead the fieldwork, almost a day's journey from Nairobi. Instead, he was going to deputize some of the Kenyan staff. Njagi was part of the strategy meeting, but the lot to make the trip fell to Joann Ambani. At a second meeting that included Hawa, a plethora of questions came up. The first one:

how to explain the research once they got there? Everybody in Kenya would have heard of HIV/AIDS, but the relatives were country people, and it might not be something they would have at the very front of their consciousness. The country cousins would be suspicious both of the disease and of medical scientists. Then there was the process of the gathering samples; it was probable none or few of them would have ever had blood taken before, and this itself would raise their suspicion and fear. "You will have to give them something in return," Hawa instructed. It could have been anything from gifts for the elders to money; she wasn't specific. Ultimately it was decided that medicine for any possible ailments would be indispensable among the gifts. "There is a lot of malaria," Hawa pointed out. "If you treat that, they will appreciate it." Joann nodded and added malaria medication to her list.

The big question though, was how to explain the actual motivation for the research; how would they justify to the people they were visiting the intricate information the scientists wanted? Why, the relatives might well want to know, were these people descending on *them* as opposed to their neighbours or anyone else and looking for AIDS? What was the connection to their sister or cousin, Hawa? The critical matter that threw the researchers into a true quandary was that Hawa's relatives did not know she was a prostitute. It seemed utterly impossible to carry out their study without somehow letting that information out of the bag. But how could they do that? Wasn't it beyond what they could possibly consider ethical? It was at this moment that Hawa herself bought decisively and definitively into the research. She was being manipulated and her privacy was being invaded not just in front of strangers from around the world, like us, but also in front of her very family. Yet she stepped up to the plate. On the matter of the explanation to her family she spoke firmly. "Leave that to me," she said.

By the time the day came to make the journey, the enterprise had ballooned into a major expedition. At six o'clock in the morning, one of the project drivers, Jackson Kinianjui, arrived at the clinic in Plummer's big white Nissan Patrol. Joann was already there, waiting with a full quotient of medical supplies, drugs, pills, sample bottles, syringes, and needles, the things she would need for her own work, plus gifts for the family. A cousin of Hawa's who wanted to tag along on the trip arrived with a suitcase, as well as with little Juma, Hawa's youngest son, in tow. While we were helping Kinianjui load everything into the four-by-four, we looked up to see Hawa herself emerge from the door of the clinic. Festooned in a billowing yellow dress, not unlike a wedding dress or something Scarlet O'Hara might have worn in *Gone with the Wind*, she sashayed out with no notion whatsoever as to how her voluminous skirt was going to be contained within the crowded vehicle. Her hair was tightly braided and she had thrown aside, for the journey to the country, her Muslim hijab. Instantly we all realized the degree to which this trip was not a chore but an event! With two vans—theirs and then, following, ours with a driver and my entire film crew—the relatives had better be ready for an inundation.

The research trip went well. Once all the samples collected made it to the lab, it fell back into the hands of MacDonald and Kaul to pick up the work. "Our job," MacDonald said, explaining the primary part of their research, "is to determine which variants the HLA specials [the resistant women with the unique combinations] possess. Is there a single mutation in their DNA?" They froze the cells of the resistant women, transported them by air freight to labs in Winnipeg and Toronto, thawed them, and then, in those North American laboratories, allowed them to continue to grow. They watched them carefully. "When we find something that appears brand new," MacDonald said, "we clone and sequence to give us something to experiment with." What their experiments showed was encouraging: the combinations and types of HLA peculiar to the resistant women stimulated the immune response to HIV better than all the others. The stoplights they operated were working.

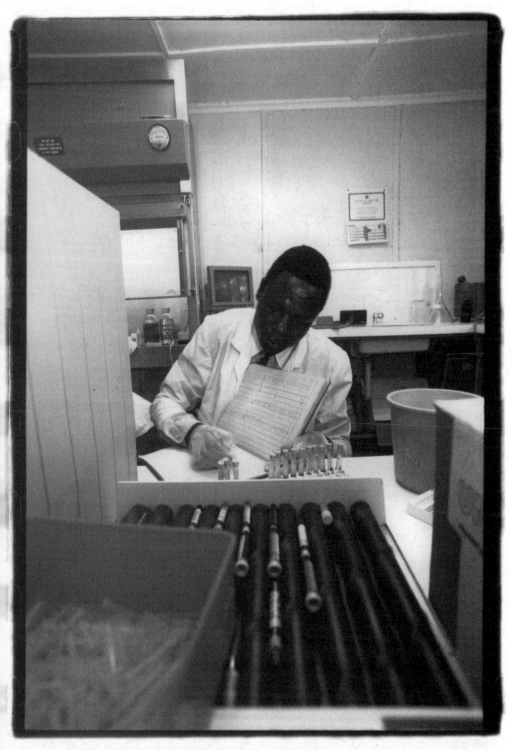

Kenyan scientist Julius Oyugi at the University of Nairobi, 1994.
PHOTO BY CHERYL ALBUQUERQUE.

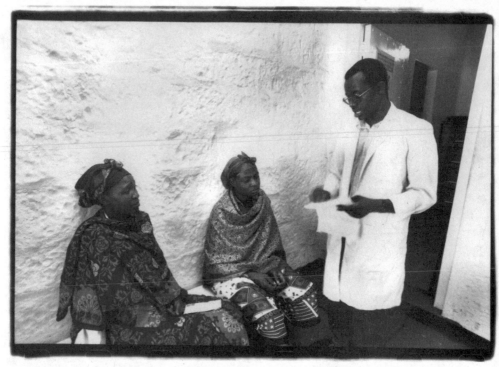

Joshua Kimani, Majengo Clinic's supervising clinician, speaks with two sex workers in the clinic's waiting room, Nairobi, 1994. PHOTO BY CHERYL ALBUQUERQUE.

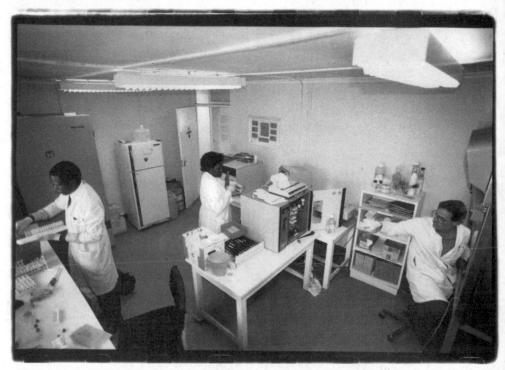

Researchers working in the Annex research lab, University of Nairobi, 1994.
FROM LEFT: Julius Oyugi, Ann Maingi, and Ian Maclean. PHOTO BY CHERYL ALBUQUERQUE.

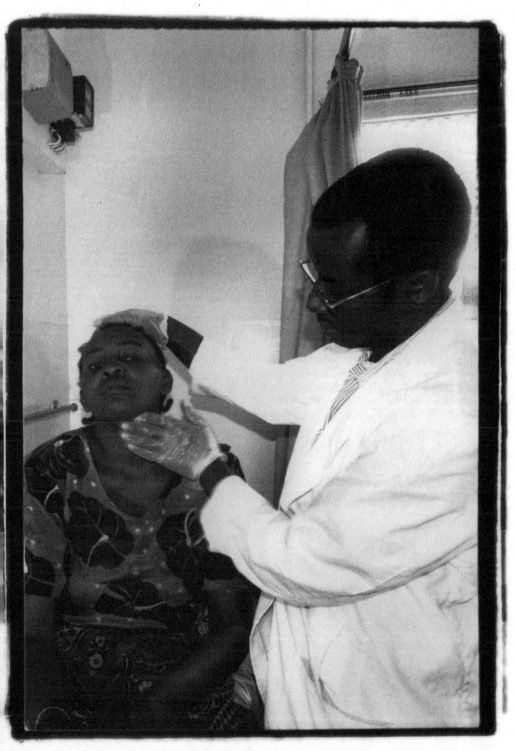

Supervising clinician Joshua Kimani performs an examination of Agnes Munyiva at the Majengo Clinic, 1994. PHOTO BY CHERYL ALBUQUERQUE.

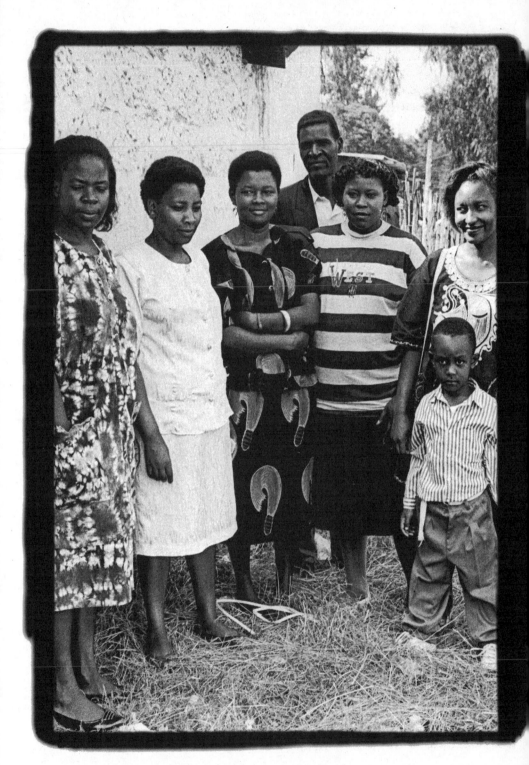

Majengo Clinic staff and family members, 1995. PHOTO BY RUPERT KAUL.

CHAPTER SIX

The Vaccine Quest;
and More Lessons From
the Immune System

A s the epidemic progressed, pressure to come up with a vaccine that
would stop HIV/AIDS in its tracks was enormous. Around the world,
countries one after the other undertook initiatives to spur their scientists to search for something that might work. Many of these enterprises were
consolidated in 1996 when the International AIDS Vaccine Initiative (IAVI) was
created as a not-for-profit, public-private partnership that put under its umbrella seventy organizations from twenty-three countries. A year later, in 1997,
the G8 leaders issued a "call for action" on HIV vaccine research.[1]

A vaccine for HIV/AIDS would have to be different than vaccines targeting
other viruses. A standard practice for protective vaccines like those for influenza, human papilloma (HPV), or chicken pox for example, is to inject a tiny
bit of virus into the human body to elicit action from the immune system de-
fences. When the real virus shows up at some later date, the body will be armed
and ready. With HIV, this strategy was not an option. No one had ever recov-
ered from AIDS. So vaccine researchers had to think about a different approach.
Another problem was something researchers were learning as the months and
years went by: this virus was a tricky, rapidly mutating one. Target one version
and, before you could blink, a new one might confront you. The vaccine search
was a challenging project.

Early on, researchers recognized that resistant sex workers who came to the
Majengo clinic might hold the key to circumventing the first of these problems.
What needed to be replicated in anybody vulnerable to HIV were the aspects
of the immune system of the resistant women, in particular their highly active

81

CT lymphocytes, which were stopping the virus from slipping into their bodies. By the late 1990s, a few scientists felt they had enough information to try to construct something.

The years 1997 and 1998 were propitious, possibly the most optimistic time in the entire history of the AIDS epidemic. After a decade and a half of global AIDS, a cure at last looked truly possible. In North America, scientists, along with the big pharmaceutical companies, were working furiously and emerging from their labs with the first versions of drug regimens that, though they would not cure the disease, promised to retard its spread through a host's body. Hope became possible for sufferers that their HIV was not necessarily a death sentence. These "triple therapies"—so named because they involved a combination of three drugs ingested daily—were complicated, still in minute supply, still being refined, still incredibly expensive. But, based on suppressants that would help people keep their T cell counts high, they promised the antiretroviral therapies that were to come. Meanwhile, there was growing hope on the vaccine front, though it was not the Canadians or Americans or Belgians who were going to take on this task, but a group from Oxford University.

Oxford had operated a medical research station in Gambia, West Africa, since the 1940s. Its purpose was to look at malaria, but also other infectious diseases. In 1990, Sarah Rowland-Jones, a scientist stationed there who was interested in HIV, took a look at the local sex worker population. She became aware of the same thing the Canadians were seeing in Nairobi: a small group in her cohort, about twenty women, were not becoming infected with the virus. She wondered if they had an immunity because of a memory of the virus from some previous exposure, perhaps long before. But she noted that six among them shared a similar HLA type, and this excited her about the possibilities of being able to trace why this was so. Follow-up was difficult because her subjects kept disappearing back to their homes, many of them not even in Gambia, but in Senegal. One day, though, she came upon Keith Fowke and Frank Plummer's publication of their findings. Immediately she got in touch, and, as she puts it, "in the spirit of collaboration, they invited us to Nairobi."[2] For the next two years, 1994 and 1995, Rowland-Jones would work out of the lab in Nairobi.[3]

Meanwhile, attention was growing all over the world around small pockets of people who appeared resistant to HIV. In addition to the resistant women, it was learned that a group of gay men in New York seemed protected. Further study determined that the good fortune these men experienced was due to a special protein that protected their cells from being infected, not only in their daily lives, but even in a lab situation. Rowland-Jones and Fowke decided to try the same test with the cells of the resistant women in their cohort, but found that in the lab they did become infected. This was in fact good news because it meant, unlike for the New Yorkers, that something immunological was protecting the women, and this made them more useful for the vaccine search.

To begin work on a vaccine, Rowland-Jones persuaded a number of researchers she had encountered in Kenya to accompany her back to Oxford.[4] Kenya was thrilled to have the project target its population. IAVI and the Wellcome Trust provided funds to set up the Kenyan AIDS Vaccine Initiative (KAVI), with upgraded labs at the University of Nairobi, and put Omu Anzala, Dr Job Bwayo, and Dr J.O. Ndinya-Achola in charge.

The vaccine was designed to stimulate the generation of cytotoxic T lymphocytes (killer T cells). At Oxford, the first animal studies and then the phase-one safety trials with forty humans (among whom a high-profile participant was Prime Minister Tony Blair) were carried out to general satisfaction. The vaccine worked on the monkeys with a 70 percent rate of creating HIV resistance and produced no harm in the humans. Kenya's job then was to prepare for the next phase of trials, assembling its own group of forty participants from the Nairobi area, all HIV-free as well as free of other diseases. The trial, which would last for about a year, would be followed by phase-two trials with people who were seen to be at a higher risk of contracting HIV. During this phase, scientists would monitor the ability of the vaccine to stimulate the immune system to defend against HIV. The phase-three trials, which would last for about three years, would determine the vaccine's absolute effectiveness in protecting a vaccinated person against the HIV/AIDS virus. As the story was publicized back home, the Kenyan press declared Bwayo, Ndinya-Achola, and Anzala "heroes."[5]

Alas, the vaccine project didn't move too far along before hitting its first bump. The British researchers took out a patent on the new vaccine in London, but failed to mention the Kenyans in the paperwork. A successful vaccine stood to make huge amounts of money, millions, possibly billions—not to mention some Nobel prizes—for its inventors. The ensuing furor was bitter. The Brits responded with lame explanations that the original DNA research was done at Oxford and that "we wanted to bar joy riders from exploiting the unpredictable circumstances in research by taking out a patent on the DNA in the vaccine."[6] They mollified the Africans by flying to Kenya and agreeing belatedly to include that country's researchers in the patent, though not as inventors of the vaccine. This was all rendered moot, however, by the fact that in the end, the vaccine didn't work. What it did with the primates in its phase-one trials, it would not do with humans. The immune response was too low and the project was shelved.

That the Oxford vaccine project, which consumed the energies of a great many people in both the U.K. and Kenya until 2005, did not pan out, was a great disappointment, especially to Kenyans who had placed all their hopes in it. Omu Anzala describes the moment when the news came that the vaccine had failed as "crushing." Walter Jaoko said, "We scientists know that an experiment can go either way, but in the general population they do not understand this, and the hopes were very high. We had to spend 2006 explaining [the failure of the vaccine] to the Kenyan people."[7]

Though few would unilaterally declare a vaccine an impossibility, failure after so much effort was sobering. Scientists did learn one thing, which was how wily a virus is HIV and how challenging the project of coming up with a vaccine to stop it. Yet none of this rendered the labours futile around trying to understand resistance. In fact, the most dogged were only emboldened. For Plummer, the research with the resistant sex workers starting to come in opened up a new, intriguing series of investigations. The way he saw it, going all the way back to Jenner, was that basic immunity had been critical to dealing with infectious diseases and understanding all manner of prevention. Therefore, the persistence of the immune-resistant women remained a critical part of the puzzle that is AIDS. The Majengo cohort of sex workers had (and still has) the advantage of being the one that has been studied for the most extensive period of time and from which has been gleaned the widest varieties of information. From 1985 through 2010, it involved 2,800 women. Two hundred new women continued to be enrolled each year, 60 percent of whom already tested positive for HIV. From enrolment on, 5 percent on average were sero-converting in every successive year. But the persistent sero-negatives were remaining stable, at about 20 percent of the total. "We have been looking at the women every which way," Plummer pointed out. "A couple of dozen similar groups have been discovered on every continent, but the Majengo women have the distinction of being observed the longest." What they had learned about resistance after all of that, he admits, is "a complexity of factors." Some of these remain consistent with a couple of centuries of study; others have proved surprising.

Keith Fowke continues to travel to Nairobi twice a year, calling the city his "second home." Along with him he brings young graduate students, the next generation of scientists for whom Fowke chairs a committee in the University of Manitoba's department of medical microbiology. A dozen or so Canadians go to Kenya each year, while, in total, ten to fifteen Kenyans have come in the other direction, to North America. Fowke's research remains focussed on the persistent sero-negative women, and his driving impetus continues to be optimism that all the work will eventually lead to some world-changing results. "As a grad student," he says, "my job was to confirm that these women were not infected and then to suggest a mechanism of how that could be confirmed, to show that they had cells that could fight off HIV. Now I focus on determining why they remain uninfected and how we might use that information to produce a vaccine."

The immune response of the HIV-resistant women was determined to have two unique characteristics. One is if they encounter an HIV-infected cell their immune systems can kill it. The other is that their immune systems are what is called "quiet." Normally, when fighting off a myriad of different infections, a person's immune system will become highly activated. HIV is certainly an infection that will activate the immune system. But as Fowke explains, you want the opposite, "you want a quiet immune system so that when your body sees a pathogen it responds to it in a very calm way. We're finding with the HIV-resistant women, compared to the other women of the cohort, that they have a very calm immune response. They're not like a car with the accelerator pushed to the floor and the engine always revving. This means they have fewer targets for HIV to infect and, when HIV is there, they will respond very quickly." The importance of understanding more about this is that whoever eventually develops a vaccine will want to stimulate an immune response, but they will not want to over-stimulate it. To learn how to achieve this is another way in which continued study of the resistant women might in the end help develop a model for vaccine production.

For his part, Plummer emphasizes that the researchers were not just learning about HIV, but about the entire immune system. As study of resistance became more and more precise and more and more detailed, he noted something he considered quite important, that in order for HIV to effectively replicate in a cell, the cell needed to be switched on. That was not the case with these women, and, again, something that made them different. "In these women, although they respond normally, the cell is not switched on. Most people don't behave like that," he said. The hypothesis of desiring a "quiet immune system" had not been considered before, and Plummer found it to be of great interest. The other positive thing, of course, was that the women remained uninfected with HIV. After twenty to twenty-five years of observation, they were still healthy. This reconfirmed for Plummer and his colleagues that whatever answer there might be to the puzzle of HIV, the kernel of it lay somewhere in the resistant women. "We have the most relevant model there is," he said. "That's very reassuring."

Reassuring, but far from satisfying in a fundamental and complete way. An ongoing frustration was that no easy answer jumped out. There is not *one* answer; the answer is not just *one thing*. When the researchers thought deeply about it, what struck them as important with the resistant women was not what part of the virus they were responding to, but how they were responding. In observing this, researchers determined that a key immune cell is something called the central memory cell, an exceedingly long-lived cell that endures in a human body for twenty to thirty years. According to Plummer, "ours, among other groups, is suggesting that that's the key cell. The current and next generation of vaccine designers must try to figure out how to get to that cell that keeps the memory of HIV with it."

The relentless pursuit of the HIV-resistant sex workers and the constant poring over the data yielded by their bodies led to a discovery that surprised the researchers. And one that also dismayed them. Rupert Kaul followed a group that took a break from the sex trade, in some cases returning to their rural villages. After a while, they returned to Nairobi and took up their old profession with their old clients. When they did so, several of them suddenly and inexplicably became infected by HIV.[8]

Kaul, after his early decision to find ways to stay on in Kenya, found himself with many opportunities to make substantial contributions and be a fully involved researcher. He met Sarah Rowland-Jones, who then invited him to her lab at Oxford. There he pursued his doctorate supervised jointly by Rowland-Jones and Plummer. In Kenya, he met other senior Canadian researchers like Stephen Moses, who introduced him to the African wilderness by taking him camping, and with whom he later collaborated on a study. Kaul would supervise a clinical trial that looked at how HIV was spread in another of Nairobi's shantytowns, the Kibera slum. He watched over more clinical trials, including one that studied whether treating STDs could be a way of slowing HIV spread. The results were inconclusive. "We were quite good at preventing STDs," he says of the results, "but we did not find that prevented HIV. A corresponding trial in Mwanza in Tanzania showed the opposite, but then a couple of trials, including one in Uganda, corresponded with ours." It left them realizing that the relationship between conventional sexually transmitted infections and HIV is complex, not as simple as originally thought. This has spawned a great deal of study and debate, with definitive answers still being sought.

When Oxford had commenced its vaccine project, Kaul had been the main link between the British university and the University of Manitoba because he was on the ground in Nairobi and in the lab at Oxford, co-supervised by scientists from each of the universities. The vaccine project involved two strands of research: the Oxford scientists had a lot of information from HIV infected people, information showing that cytotoxic T lymphocytes were important in control of HIV if you were infected. (CTLs, also known as killer T cells belong to a sub-group of T lymphocytes, a type of white blood cell, that are capable of inducing the death of infected somatic or tumor cells; they kill cells that are infected with viruses.) The Manitoba researchers found that they could pick up CTLs of low frequency in people who were exposed but not infected. The combination of these strains of research led them to the premise that a vaccine that could induce CTLs might be important in protecting against HIV.

Now a clinician-scientist with his own lab specializing in HIV at the University of Toronto, Kaul sees patients in Toronto and also when he travels to Nairobi, a trip he continues to make. He maintains his collaboration with the University of Nairobi and University of Manitoba, continuing research into the peculiarities of the persistent HIV-negative women and working with Plummer to continue to look at resistance from all sorts of vantage points. Kaul's task is one aspect of this work: immune responses in the genital tract. His specialty is relations between co-infections and HIV, asking questions such as why other STDs do in fact make it more likely for a person to get HIV, or why the clinical trials might not have worked in preventing HIV. In observing the Majengo cohort, he has noted how many of the resistant women have other STDs such as herpes.[9]

Kaul was the kind of researcher who fit, for Plummer, into the group of young people he hoped would come along to keep the collaboration going into the next generation. "I was always happy," Plummer says, "to have people willing to ask fresh questions." This new generation were clinicians as well as scientists. Richard Lester, born in Smithers B.C. and a graduate of the University of Alberta, initiated a program whereby health-care workers use cell phones to keep in touch with their far-flung patients, usually to remind them to take their medications, including the vital antiretroviral pills that need to be ingested regularly every day. After decades of enduring expensive and exceedingly haphazard telephone service, the cell phone revolution has placed a mobile phone into the hands of almost every Kenyan, even the most impoverished shantytown dweller. Putting these at the service of people's health care is proving to be equally revolutionary. For his part, Rupert Kaul also has been deeply involved with the Majengo clinic's supervising clinician, Dr Joshua Kimani, in the rollout of antiretroviral therapies now available to all HIV-infected women who are part of the clinic cohort, and with an initiative called the Sex Worker Outreach Program (SWOP) on River Road in downtown Nairobi. As they do this, they seek answers to their ever-more pointed questions. Since sex workers are a major way HIV spreads into the general population, will treating them with antiretroviral therapies reduce HIV transmission? Sex workers have lots of infections, so even if you're being treated might not there be HIV still present in the genital tract? If that's the case, says Kaul, "what's the effect of going on ARV treatment? We're looking at studies that try to explain that to us."

Then, of course, there is the matter of the women who took a break and then, after their period of immune quiescence, became infected with HIV. Rupert Kaul continues to study eleven of these women. For Plummer, it was a great shock to discover, as he puts it, "women who have been uninfected for ten years and then suddenly become infected." But for a scientist, a shock is usually just a signal to refocus research. "What changes?" he asks. "The commonalities were that women who sero-converted very late had recently taken a break from sex work. I'm now following a hypothesis that the immune system needs the constant stimulation of seeing HIV in order to keep the subjects resistant. In a paradoxical way this reinforces the hypothesis that it's an acquired immunity, they have to be exposed to it consistently." According to Plummer, the phenomenon also reveals that resistance is not something genetic; nobody has a gene that makes you resistant (though there is clustering in families, connected probably to common HLA types). The lesson for the individual resistant sex worker: don't take a break, or if you do, take a permanent break.

Another group they watch are women whose commonality is that they are "non-progressors." These are women who are known to be infected with HIV, but who go for a very long time without showing any symptoms of becoming ill with AIDS. Even without antiretroviral treatment they don't get sick. Plummer understands that all over the world they are finding a few people with HIV that doesn't progress, who seem able to control their HIV. These, he claims, are very interesting to him. So the Nairobi collaboration continues to watch two groups: people who are exposed but don't get infected and people who get infected, but for whom the disease does not progress. They have also established along the way that HIV resistance is marked by gene traits consistent with people with diabetes. The frustration, or at least the challenge, continues to be, as it has been for a long time: conventional approaches to vaccine development have not worked, necessitating other approaches.

In a Toronto *Globe and Mail* article, Frank Plummer told reporter Graeme Smith that he likes to take the detective approach to his research.[10] "You can't just slash somebody open to find out what's wrong," he said. "It's a detective approach. I liked that." Fifteen years after identifying women who appeared resistant to HIV, the ongoing labours are still oriented toward identifying the key components that make those women—or anybody—resistant. To do this, the scientists are patiently studying every possible gene, getting a picture of the genetic signature of the resistant women, getting an idea of pathways. "If we can stimulate or inhibit pathways," posits Plummer, "that would make an important contribution to a vaccine. Our group has made a great contribution to understanding in the field of HIV resistance. Our next contribution is that we may not develop an HIV vaccine itself, but we can inform the vaccine developers how you want the immune system to respond to that vaccine. Do you want to produce antibodies against HIV or do you want to produce this type of cell or that type of cell? What is the protective mechanism is really what our greatest contribution can be."

CHAPTER SEVEN

The Kenyan Side: Squaring the Collaboration

F amau Ali is a middle-aged man with a tan complexion and frizzy, black
hair starting to grey. He wears a khaki shirt enhanced with epaulets, creating the impression of a uniform and some accompanying authority,
though not a crisp, on-parade uniform, and so not a terribly imposing authority.
When we met, he was squashed into the corner of an old couch in an office at the
Majengo clinic, snuggled against his twelve-year-old son—who was suffering
that morning from the sniffles. On the other end of the couch loomed a stack
of papers, reports, and other various documents spilled over from the filing
cabinets of a busy and overcrowded surgery. The office, as well as overflow for
papers and a meeting room for interviews, doubles as lunch room for the staff
whenever they can get a minute from their incessant duties. But at the moment
there was only Famau, his son, and me. Famau Ali is assistant chief of the Pumwani community and chairman of the village health committee, a post he has
held for some time and in which capacity he participated in approving the use of
the Majengo clinic by the HIV collaborators. He took part in welcoming them
after they got that approval and has kept an eye on things ever since.

That Ali should be a judge of the relationship between the outsider medical
scientists and the local people of Kenya might seem arbitrary. But then why not?
In some sense he represents all ordinary Kenyans, bystanders—though not really—to all that was going on in their country throughout its battle with AIDS.
The good thing about the relationship with the scientists, he stated, was the educational aspect. "The program here convinced the sex workers to reduce their
diseases. Which is important; they are our mothers," he said. What he and others
liked less, that which even grated on some of them, was a sense that they were not

given sufficient credit for how important the Kenyan story became to the world outside. They were objects in something they knew to be overwhelmingly large, but that they didn't quite understand. "We are guinea pigs; we have sacrificed to the whole world," Ali told me in a manner not so much complaining as resigned.

Ali was deeply disappointed when the vaccine that Oxford University, along with KAVI, worked on with so much fanfare did not materialize. Kenyans had been led to believe it would succeed, and that would have been a great moment for the people of Pumwani-Majengo. They have had to recover from the letdown. On a material level, he declares, their rewards have been modest: the council office received a television set from Frank Plummer that they claim to use for educational purposes. But Ali periodically dreamed of much more: that there would be scholarships for shantytown children to go to school, that there would be "economic development." He pushed for grant applications to be made to CIDA, he claims, but nothing came of this. He said everybody was disappointed when Plummer left in 2000 to return to Canada to take on his new job as chief of the Canadian government's new national laboratory in Winnipeg. "He had a big job to go to in Canada, bigger than us," Ali said. Yet in conclusion he confirmed, "We still appreciate what the universities have done."

If Ali seemed a bit grudging in his evaluation, others were not. Outside, under the shade of a new tent and awning supplied by Bill Gates's foundation to enlarge the waiting area of the clinic, now that one of its big tasks is supplying HIV-positive women with their regular doses of antiretroviral therapies, four women gathered on plastic chairs. Hawa Chelangat, who is number 935 in the clinic roster; Rosemary John, who is 602; Leolalida Maliseli, 058; and Josephine Kokumbaza, 005. In 2010, these women were the senior members of the cohort, the oldest survivors, and, of course, the cream of the persistent negatives. Arriving for our meeting, they looked the part, like senior ladies at the church bazaar. Rosemary showed up in a pink dress and white pearls. When the conversation began, it was not about sex work, but about grandchildren. Hawa now has four. Rosemary has seven children and eighteen grandchildren. Leolalida has four grandchildren. Josephine, who arrived late, has eight grandchildren. This information, not strictly on the topic of the meeting, nevertheless served a substantial purpose; it placed everything in a context of not the exotic, but of normal life. The swapping of stories about these women's grandchildren was a significant reminder of what was cut short by the awful epidemic in so many families and for all those mothers who never got to reach the stage of becoming grandmothers.

Eventually, the talk did get around to HIV/AIDS, the common bond that had tied the group for so many years to this clinic. This, of course, brought up memories of those not so fortunate to last long enough for antiretroviral therapies to come along—those who died. The women spoke respectfully about some of the names on that list. They also told how Elizabeth Ngugi early on tried to warn them, "get out of this job or you'll be dead." "There was no medicine then," they reiterated, referring to the therapies that now keep people alive. They kept working, though to a person they claim that they became more dedicated to using condoms. Though, again, none of them used them all the time. They tried, but could think of very few colleagues who had given up sex work and said that they themselves kept working because they needed to feed their children. What else was there to do? And they watched their friends die. The women resolutely resisted complaining to a visitor. They offered stories instead about how clinic medicine cured their children's illnesses. They did venture some initiatives in support of their own rights: at one point they asked for a 100 KSh increase (about $1.30 CDN) in the stipend given them when they provided blood. They also recalled not liking one of the clinicians who was briefly in charge of the clinic. "He was not a good doctor," they claimed, and, in response to their concerns, the offensive doctor was removed. This sense of their own power pleased them.

Collaboration is a nice, friendly term—like cooperation—assuming all the best forms of common goals and common cause. In substantial part, the Nairobi collaboration embodied this definition. It was, more strikingly, however, a mingle of exceedingly different people from very different worlds. If you looked at all the players, their backgrounds, assumptions, opportunities in life, you could not have gathered together a group more divergent, more different, one to the next. At one extreme was a doctor, born in a small city in Canada where snow lay on the ground for half the year; at the other, a sex worker from Nairobi, just south of the equator, where there was never even frost. The doctor was highly educated, with several medical degrees; behind him were enormous resources, both of his university institution and of the granting agencies of his government. He enjoyed lofty status in his community and could come and go at will to meetings and conferences anywhere in the world, staying at fine hotels. The sex worker had three years of formal education in a school without electricity in rural Kenya. The extent of her travels were 300-kilometre bus rides between her rural village and the city of Nairobi. The doctor spoke English and was Christian. The sex worker spoke Swahili and was a Muslim. The doctor and his family had the resources to live in material comfort both in Nairobi and in

Canada; the jerry-built shanty in which the sex worker and her children slept every night would fit twice over inside most North American garages.

That Frank Plummer and Hawa Chelangat ended up as two links of an intense partnership is one of the truly extraordinary aspects of the world we live in. Occupying the space between them, of course, were myriad others representing every class and interest, both Western and African. There were well-off and educated Kenyans—as well as those young and hungry and eager to make their mark. Among the Europeans and North Americans were some who were interested purely in the abstractions of science; others in occupying the front lines to attend to the sick. Some were out to solve riddles; others to save the world. Could the tenuous fabric of a broadly based collaboration serve to connect such a diverse group? It seemed a great challenge to all sides of the Nairobi collaboration to understand one another's positions completely, and a far reach to believe that what was good for any one of them would be automatically—and consistently—good for all the others. There was always the potential for extraordinary connection, with people who would otherwise never meet working shoulder to shoulder. But inside was the persistent potential for divergence.

A relationship between the project and the community of Majengo sex workers was indispensable for the path the research was taking. And though it was generally a good relationship, it would not always be an easy one. Central to it was a fundamental contradiction. As the senior women had declared when they gathered to reflect on the project, there were many things about which they were happy. Foremost here was health care for themselves and their children in a community that would have a difficult time obtaining affordable and reliable care under any other circumstances. The project also provided community: the clinic became a clubhouse where the women could gather to gossip and reliably encounter their friends. From time to time the parking lot inside its gates would get cleared for a giant party with fire pits dug, meat braised, huge pots of rice and vegetables cooked. The women had an organization, encouraged by Elizabeth Ngugi, and attempts were made over the years to get funding for initiatives that would better their lives. With a grant from CIDA, Ngugi had in fact arranged training for 120 women so they could move out of the sex trade. Two-thirds of the enrollees reportedly succeeded. But the fundamental contradiction kept coming back to haunt both the women and the project's researchers. If the women did not continue as sex workers in the low-end shantytown environment, there could be no research. It would grind to a halt. Or, the researchers would have to go somewhere else and try to set up all over again. The Majengo shantytown sex-worker clinic was an ideal laboratory, and it needed the women as much if not more than they needed it. Famau Ali had called them "guinea pigs," and though that might seem an indecorous terminology, it was, in some sense, what they were.

This tension reached a head in early 2006 when Toronto *Globe and Mail* correspondent Stephanie Nolen wrote a feature story under the lurid headline, "Sex Slaves For Science." Nolen was a seasoned and award-winning writer, having lived for years in Johannesburg. Her story from the Majengo shantytown featured one of the longest enrolled of the resistant sex workers, a woman named Salome Simon. Though the article filled out the story of the discovery that the small cohort of sex workers were resistant and quoted various of the scientists about what that might mean and where they were heading with their work, the memorable point of the story—enhanced by the headline—was about an imbalance. The scientists had become successful and well-known around the world, the University of Manitoba had over the years received $23 million in grants; the Bill and Melinda Gates Foundation grant for $9.2 million had just been awarded; the University of Nairobi medical school campus was just about to receive its new $3.8 million laboratory. But Salome Simon still worked twelve hours a day servicing clients and had nothing to show for her career but "a couple of kangas, the bright print wraps she wears as skirts, and a couple of blouses. A transistor radio, some aluminum pots, and one little luxury, a gilded bottle of spicy perfume." All those millions, the story reported, and yet Simon still has sex for eighty cents in a fly-filled, mud-walled room. "With no sex workers, what would happen to their research?" the article asked.[1]

The story incensed the Canadians, particularly Frank Plummer. The day after it appeared, he fired off an e-mail to Nolen charging that "through a bad headline, selective reporting and facile analysis your article has sullied twenty years of ground breaking work on finding solutions to the immense problem of HIV and as a spinoff the prevention of many tens of thousands of HIV infections in Kenya and elsewhere. Hopefully the damage will be short lived." Then he went on to turn the tables on the Africa-based journalist. "I would ask you to look in the mirror. As someone who is making they're [sic] living and reputation off the misery of Africa what are YOU or the Globe doing about it. Your answer will be that you are reporting it and that alleviating poverty or getting women out of sex work is beyond you. You can write about it but not much more."

Larry Gelmon, from his office overseeing the project in Nairobi, weighed in with his own missive to the unfortunate Nolen, picking out the "Sex Slave" headline (that she herself claimed to be appalled by): "Most unfortunate is the headline and the implications that there may have been exploitation of the sex worker cohorts by the Univ. Manitoba researchers. You discuss some of the arguments for and against this within the article, but the sensationalist and inaccurate headline (what justification is there for use of the word 'slaves'?) distorts the content of the article for the majority of readers who would not have read the whole, and also demeans the high-quality reporting."

Behind all aspects of the Nairobi collaboration—indeed behind all relationships between Western actors and the developing world—lurked the image of a kind of selflessness and purity. What could be more noble than medical science saving lives and setting out to save an entire continent? This narrative was the one offered back home to both funders and the general public. It was also the ethic justifying whatever sacrifices many of the researchers might have felt they were making in everything from earnings to energy to family. But the high-minded notion went only so far. Few things in the real world can continue within such a consistent frame, certainly not over the length of time that this collaboration lasted. No matter how hard you might work at defusing them, contradictions are inherent.

It was always a delicate business to engineer such a coming together of partners and call it a collaboration. The participants were from different parts of the world, from different backgrounds, and (sometimes) with different agendas. The power imbalance was not a fantasy but a reality best illustrated by the fact that the North Americans and Europeans could come and go at will. When they wanted to be back home at their own universities doing other things, that's where they were. The imbalance was built in, and it was soon realized by most everybody that the project could only function when that disparity was acknowledged as the reality under which everybody worked. The very best moments of the thirty-year collaboration are remembered as those times when both sides have brought their strengths and their gifts toward a common objective and then have grown together. The objective hasn't *always* been common, but that the collaboration has lasted and thrived speaks to the fact that the sharing has gone in both directions.

Where things seemed to work very well for both the Westerners and the Kenyans was at the professional level. There were Kenyan professionals who embraced the objectives of the collaboration, who were vital to both clinical and research success, and who (some of them) got substantial parts of their education as a result of it. Omu Anzala received his PhD at the University of Manitoba; Joshua Kimani and J.O. Ndinya-Achola went to the University of Washington to study for their master's of public health, as did Kawango Agot. Julius Oyugi studied at the University of Manitoba as well as at Oxford. Walter Joako likewise studied at Oxford. These all went on to occupy high-level positions both in the Nairobi and Kenyan health system, and inside the collaboration. Anzala, Ndinya-Achola, and Jaoko all became chairs of the University of Nairobi medical microbiology department; Kimani became chief clinician for the collaboration; Agot was manager of the UNIM (universities of Nairobi, Illinois, and Manitoba) circumcision project in Kisumu.

Countless others, equally important, spent most of their days unsung, save that the collaboration was central to their working lives and their skills and labours were critical to it. Numerous of these were among the 400 gathered at the January 2010 meeting at the Mayfair Court Hotel, filling the conference halls to either present the details of the work they were doing or take in the information provided by others. They were people like John Mungai, who spent each and every day meticulously and patiently counselling men and women about to get their AIDS tests at the Baba Dogo clinic on the far side of town, or Sophie Wacharo, his colleague who gave half an hour of her time to demonstrate for me how the new HIV rapid tests operated. They were people like Erastus Muthoga, for almost twenty years a technician in the laboratory at the University of Nairobi, lately put in charge of the shiny new machinery of the Level 3 lab, who proudly proclaimed, "If there s a catastrophe, we will handle it."

On the ground, scientific research, not unlike almost any other foreign-sponsored venture, is supported by a vast army of locals who are not professionals but without whom nothing would work. For the Nairobi project, these included secretaries, cleaners, receptionists, basic lab workers, and people like the drivers. One of these is Jackson Kinyanjui, steady as the day is long and with an intelligent broad face. Kinyanjui was twenty-four years old when he came to the attention of Frank Plummer in 1994, pitched as a serious young man with no bad habits who knew cars, having been a driver for a tourist outfitter, a job that took him into all the back corners of Kenya. Soon he was living on the Plummer property and serving as Frank's personal driver. Unlike almost every foreigner with status or responsibility in Nairobi, Plummer had never until that moment had a driver. Having one, he soon learned, made a great difference to his life. A driver, in the culture of postcolonial Kenya, is more than just someone who drives a car, but is best understood in terms of the old colonial Kenya. A driver is like a valet in an old English movie; he knows everything about his employer and is unstintingly loyal—not just professionally loyal, but emotionally loyal.

But what both the Westerners and more specifically the Kenyans wanted out of their collaboration—along with combatting the scourge of HIV/AIDS—was something called "capacity growth." This, cited repeatedly in statements of purpose and speeches given to one another by both the foreigners and the Kenyans, centred around the medical personnel. All the expended energy and effort had to lead to a contingent, especially within the University of Nairobi, of scientists and teachers, doctors and researchers who were more able, more competent, more independent, more confident than their predecessors might have been a generation before. This was a goal both stated and implied. And to some degree it came to fruition. A number of the young professional medical people who were mentored within the collaboration actually *became* the collaboration in due time, and this is what players on both sides cite among their proudest achievements. A good example is Joshua Kimani. Now in his mid-forties, bright, ambitious, and exceedingly dedicated—yet retaining a youthful energetic step— Kimani was, in 1987, a third-year medical student. One morning, a Canadian with curly, brown hair came to lecture his class on the topic of sexually transmitted diseases. The visiting white man was Frank Plummer. "HIV had just come," Kimani recalls. "People didn't really understand it, and talked about it in only the most abstract manner. Frank, though, believed that STDs had a link with this new infection everybody was talking about."

At the end of term, Kimani and his fellow student and pal, Ephantus Njagi, sought out Plummer and volunteered to spend their holiday working at the clinic he had talked about in the Majengo shantytown. Their offer accepted, they went to Majengo, where, trundling every day out to the clinic, they got to know the community of sex workers who were the clinic's clients, observed sample collection, did lab rotations, and learned to do the ELISA test to determine HIV status. In June of 1989, at the closing of their fourth year, both Kimani and Njagi chose infectious diseases as their elective. They were rewarded when the University of Manitoba sent air tickets to take them to spend the months of July, August, and September in Winnipeg. There the young students met people who were their contemporaries, like Keith Fowke, and senior colleagues like Robert Brunham, Joanne Embree, and Allan Ronald, who were by now well-known members of the collaboration with their names on numerous research papers. The awestruck young men were invited to do rounds in Winnipeg hospitals and rub shoulders with more Canadian counterparts. "By the time we came back home," Kimani recalls, "we had seen a different world, and been opened up to the opportunities in public health."

The experience was transformative. His fifth-year advisor at the University of Nairobi tried to get Kimani to select internal medicine as his specialty. "Who cares about HIV?" he asked. "There will be no money in that, it's a poor people's disease." But Kimani resisted the overtures. "I wanted to talk about current things, not just textbooks," he says. "I wanted room to think outside the box; to be confronted with problems and then have to find solutions." To the young Kenyan doctors like Kimani and Njagi, Frank Plummer represented the novel way of doing things. As well, he was a "cool guy" in their eyes. One of the first things Kimani noticed was that Plummer had a nice car, a Subaru with a digital odometer. "The conventional wisdom in Kenya and in the medical school was that if you follow public health, you'll die poor. Frank contradicted this. These guys didn't look like they were suffering."

Infectious diseases, particularly HIV/AIDS—in the context of public health— looked like a deeply interesting and challenging choice. In retrospect, Kimani puts it, "We took a calculated risk to look outside the Kenyan prism." And the more they entered into that world, the more sure they became that it was a good choice—not just for the good they could do, the challenging work they would encounter, but also for the opportunities it afforded for their personal experience and growth. The Canadians encouraged Kimani and other members of the up-and-coming generation of young Kenyans. "Whenever Ronald came to Nairobi he would take the students to lunch; Frank would take them to the Burger Chef in Hurlingham. He became our mentor without knowing it," says Kimani. Soon Kimani was off to Sweden with colleagues in the "physicians against nuclear war" movement. Then, in the mid-1990s, the University of Washington accepted him to study for a master's in public health. Fifteen years later, Kimani is clinical director of the University of Manitoba/Nairobi Collaborative Research Group, overseeing four shantytown clinics and another for sex workers in the middle of the city.

Another recruit through an almost accidental meeting was Omu Anzala. In 1988, Anzala, a recently graduated doctor, held the position of medical officer in the district hospital at Kapsabet, a farming town of 15,000 people in the Rift Valley a couple of hours northwest of Nairobi. One day, Frank Plummer showed up to talk to the staff of the district hospital about sexually transmitted diseases. Afterwards, the young doctor Anzala approached him expressing an interest in the whole field of infectious diseases. Plummer suggested he head to Nairobi and have a chat with the people at the medical school. He did so, encountering the chair of the microbiology department, Hannington Pamba, who encouraged him to join the department and apply to become a tutorial fellow. Anzala did this, too, then looked up Plummer again and got himself posted to the Majengo clinic, as the second Kenyan doctor to work there. This was 1989.

From there, things in his career zoomed full-speed forward. In 1990, he received a CIDA scholarship to go to Canada to get his master's degree in microbiology. He arrived in Winnipeg in October 1991, and spent the winter freezing as he waited for buses to take him from his downtown lodgings to his classes at the university campus. "I got myself a huge stuffy parka coat," he recalls, which apparently he never took off. "When I was indoors," he says, "I would sweat like crazy. But then as soon as I stepped out of doors, all that sweat would turn to ice." Though Allan Ronald, he recalls, urged him to pursue public health, he wanted to do more basic science. And that's what he did.

Despite the challenges of a cold climate, Anzala stayed on in Winnipeg until 1996, completing his PhD at the University of Manitoba. Then he went to another chilly country, the U.K., where he had been awarded a post-doctoral fellowship at Oxford under the supervision of Sarah Rowland-Jones. He joined the collaboration around the AIDS vaccine, his experience rounded out as Kenya beckoned him back, placing him in charge of KAVI, which was the local partner for the Oxford University project. In 2010, Omu Anzala became chair of medical microbiology at the University of Nairobi.

By taking this role, Anzala brought the Nairobi collaboration full circle. Recruited and trained by Westerners almost in equal measure to his being recruited and trained by Kenyans, he was, at least through the breadth of his experience and education, a sort of hybrid: a little DNA from both sides. But would he (and others) become a novel species of trans-global internationalist scientist for whom borders and passports were just formalities, or would he need to choose, at some point, more parochial loyalties? When he became chair, Anzala joined a list of previous chairs, each of whom, for their time in office, formally represented the Kenyan side of the collaboration. Though for the most part—and certainly on the surface—there was considerable common cause shared by the two sides, foreign and Kenyan, maintaining a perfect balance was never easy. Robert Brunham, head of the University of Manitoba department of medical microbiology for twelve years from 1988 to 1999, dealt with three chairs on the University of Nairobi side, "each," he says, "with different goals." Nsanze, Pamba, Wamola, Ndinya-Achola, Bwayo, Joako, Anzala: these men (and the department heads were always men) had their own difficult job, juggling a relationship with the foreigners all the while upholding what was deemed good for both the University of Nairobi and their country. These were not always, of course, the same thing. During Brunham's time, when Isaac Wamola followed J.O. Ndinya-Achola, and then Job Bwayo followed him, the emphasis for the Kenyans shifted from what Brunham recalls as "a purely collegial collaboration bent on solving scientific problems," to one more loaded with politics. By this time, Kenya was gaining confidence both in its abilities and in its obligations to tackle its own problems. "Capacity building for Africans," Brunham noted, took precedence; the operative question, posed perpetually, was "How does this benefit Kenya?" Pressure built to have things show that the University of Nairobi was leading the collaboration, even though the money was still coming from across the ocean. It was, admits Brunham, "tricky."

In the lore of the project, certain characterizations have persisted. Job Bwayo held senior posts both at the university and KEMRI, all the while overseeing important research.[2] But he was roundly seen by the foreigners as "difficult." Isaac Wamola had a reputation for excessively following the letter of the law. Joanne Embree still recalls him as "absolutely terrified of what we were going to do." "We" being the North Americans and Europeans who, she believed, he and possibly other high-level Kenyans perceived as "a bunch of uncontrolled university professors from another country whose goal is science—and personal advancement in science—and who are not Kenyan." Does this mean that what might be understood from the Kenyan side as a natural progression was not always easy for the outsiders? To some degree, it appears so. Little plays of power, some of them petty, got enacted as each side tried to remind the other of their place. The foreigners, on occasion, found themselves biding their time while Kenyan officials stalled in signing such things as letters permitting scientific samples to leave the country. An oft-repeated story is about the documents necessary to allow a promising young Canadian researcher, Jacques Pepin, to get to work languishing on the University of Nairobi microbiology department chairman's desk. So much time passed that Pepin packed up and departed Kenya in frustration.

All in all, though, "difficult" is not how the grand span of the relationship is thought of by most who participated over the years. Most, on both sides, expanded their learning and experience, and developed friendships they would never have had the opportunity for in any other kind of world. Working together and learning together was a leveller far more than it was a barrier. The common cause of a hugely challenging project turned everybody into a sort of family. The idea of the team, the idea of collaboration, in the end, was a necessity; the dynamics of a complicated enterprise could not have progressed in any other way. There needed to be trust, there needed to be both sharing and delegating of authority. As Joshua Kimani expressed it: "In research, you need networks. One person cannot be an expert in everything. If one partner is not good at immunology, you have to reach out to friendly partners who can bring their expertise to the table." This is fundamentally how things came to be over thirty years, and the bumps of differences, while needing to be acknowledged, were, for the most part, simply that: bumps.

One of the first things you see when you enter the lobby of the University of Manitoba/Nairobi Collaboration laboratory building is a row of framed photographs mounted on a wall above the reception desk. Five serious looking, youthful, intense faces. The photo gallery is a shrine to the memory of young Kenyans, all participants in the collaboration, all dead in an afternoon.

On December 14, 1995, a convoy of vehicles carried twenty-six project members—including Frank Plummer, Allan Ronald, and Stephen Moses—from an AIDS conference in Kampala Uganda. This was an important regional conference, and Frank Plummer wanted his staff to attend. It had ended on a successful note, everybody agreeing there had been ample shared information and fertile new ideas. People commenced the return home in a buoyant mood knowing that, once they got back to Nairobi, the next thing on the agenda would be the Christmas break.

The problem with the trip home was that December is the season of the short rains, and, just across the border into Kenya, the vehicles and drivers entered a blinding rainstorm. It was three o'clock in the afternoon. Three of the cars, coping with bad visibility and bad orientation, took a wrong turn. They soon realized their mistake, turned around and headed back toward the main road. But, at this point, the lead car was hit head-on by an oncoming truck. Five people were in the car: the driver, Edward Oyugi; three senior research physicians, James Nasio, Patrick Nyange, and Tom Obongo; and administrative manager Ruth Auma.

Within five minutes a car bearing Ronald and Moses came upon the carnage, and realized right away that the mangled vehicle was one of theirs. Police were already present at the scene, as was a crowd of about a hundred bystanders. In those brief moments, awful things had already happened. Passports and money had already been stolen from the bodies of the dead and injured. Some of the car's occupants were clearly dead, but Ruth Auma was still alive. An ambulance finally arrived to take her to the hospital in Nakuru, the closest big town. Ronald and Moses jumped into their car to follow, knowing that when they got to Nakuru they would have to telephone Frank Plummer who, in a vehicle near the head of the convoy, would already be home in Nairobi.

The situation in Nakuru was disheartening. Doctors in the hospital there had little to work with; there was no blood available for transfusion and no imaging equipment. They were unable to save Auma. Ruth Auma was thirty-seven and the mother of two teenaged children. She had been with the project for eleven years, including two spent in Winnipeg, where she had undertaken management training. James Nasio was a skilled clinical physician who had worked in the Majengo clinic and had been to Seattle for training at the University of Washington, as had Patrick Nyange. It was a terrible loss that took a long time to heal.

CHAPTER EIGHT

An Experiment in Kisumu

D ecember 2004. The Kenya Airways evening flight from Nairobi banked into the final phase of its steep descent. Pressing my face to the port-hole window I could see a swirl of blue-green waters: Lake Victoria, the second-largest freshwater lake in the world, the fabled environs of King Ru-manika and explorers Burton and Speke. The lake circumnavigated in a canoe by Henry Morton Stanley, who was looking to see if any part of it emptied out to become the Nile. Then all of a sudden we were past the water and it was all palm trees and elephant grass as the little plane levelled in toward the runway, delivering, at precisely 7 p.m., its twenty passengers to the small Kisumu airport. Minutes later, waiting on the damp tarmac for the luggage to be brought round on the wire-sided wagon pushed by the baggage handlers, I looked about to see if there might be a taxi. Almost instantly, a smiling young man approached. He asked if I needed a ride, then led me to where a fleet of sagging cars, none of them with taxi markings, was parked. Each had a staff of two, the driver and the tout. Mine introduced himself, "Moses," and his partner, "Johnson." Moses Onyango and Ochanga Johnson, with me in the backseat, set off for the ten-minute trip to town. It had rained, leaving puddles in the road, and everything a verdant green. In the gathering dusk, cows grazed in the ditches and we passed people on bicycles.

"Are you with an NGO?" Moses turned in his seat and posed what was prob-ably the inevitable question for the newly arrived white person. "No," I answered, "but I'm visiting one. UNIM." I caught myself being slightly hesitant. I wondered whether UNIM might not be a bit controversial locally. The idea behind it was to test a hypothesis that circumcision of young males would affect HIV rates—for the better—and to do that, persuading a great number of young Kisumu men, men like

Moses and Johnson, to get circumcised. "Do you know them?" I asked. "Oh yes," Moses answered. "We know Bob, we know Kawango. Sometimes we drive them."

They drove me to a place called the Nyanza Club, depositing me at the front gate and helping with my bag. "You will want to go to the clinic tomorrow," Moses stated. "What time will we pick you up?" In my mind I had settled on an alternate plan for getting to the clinic, which was about four kilometres away on the other side of town. On a previous visit I'd worked out what I considered a perfect local transportation strategy: a fairly agreeable walk past government buildings and park-like gardens for the first part of the trip until I reached the edge of downtown. Then all I had to do was flag down a bicycle taxi, locally called *boda-boda*, climb on the extended seat behind the cyclist, and get the rest of the trip for a cost of about twenty-five cents. I was intending to do that now, rather than shell out seven to ten dollars for the car taxi. Yet I could hardly refuse these friendly fellows. "Alright," I agreed, "pick me up at nine." I gave Johnson a business card so he would remember my name.

At nine o'clock the next morning, with the sun already becoming hot, I walked up to the front gate to wait for my promised taxi. It didn't come. I asked the guard if he knew Johnson and Moses and had they been round. "Not yet," he said. I decided to give them five minutes. It was Saturday, and the clinic would only be open for the morning and then closed until Monday. I didn't want to waste the precious hours. After five minutes I set off on foot, muttering a few complaints about the unreliability of a couple of drivers from whom I expected better; my old plan would have to be activated after all. But then I calmed down. Under the shade of the great trees that spread across the road the walk was pleasant. I passed the inevitable grazing cows and the whitewashed walls fronting the provincial government buildings. The Kenyan flag flapped dutifully in the breeze. Two workers with machetes were cutting grass on the boulevard, chopping away rhythmically with steady, arching swings. Using my passing as an excuse, they took a break and waved. Suddenly a banged-up grey Peugeot pulled up beside me. I didn't recognize the driver who held up a small white card. "Is this you, Mr Larry?" he asked. It was my business card. "Johnson and Moses are very sorry," he said. "Their car has broken down and it will take until afternoon to repair it. They have sent me to find you."

The UNIM clinic was situated in a compound that was on the verge of achieving a sort of critical mass in terms of health-care activities. Next door was a municipal clinic, newly fixed up where, on this morning city food workers were lined up for their monthly cholera tests. At the end of the parking lot, new construction was underway on two more buildings that would join the municipal clinic and UNIM with their own undertakings, both in the field of HIV research. The UNIM clinic was smart and stylish, nicely designed of gleaming white stucco with the clinic logo painted in bright blue. Across the fence was a private girls' school that suffered by comparison. Constructed in 2001, the clinic had doubled in size after an addition in 2002. Inside was a spacious waiting room filled already that morning with about twenty-five young men. In one direction were consulting rooms and the surgery; in the other a file storage room and a fully operational lab. Upstairs were offices, a conference room, and a data processing centre. I asked for Kawango, one of the people mentioned by Moses on the taxi ride the night before, and was directed to an office next to the lab. A tall, cheerful woman wearing an African print outfit and sporting horn-rim glasses greeted me.

Kawango Agot was a Kisumu local. She had left Kenya as a young woman to study in America and came back with a PhD in medical geography from the University of Washington. For her thesis, she'd returned to her roots and done something that turned out to help immensely in her interview for this job: she'd undertaken a study of circumcision in the Kisumu area. On her desk was a well-thumbed Bible and a cell phone which, when it rang, burbled "Waltzing Mathilda." As clinic manager, she was in charge of hiring all the local staff, more than forty of them, including the surgeons who performed the circumcisions on through to counsellors, lab staff, recruiters, drivers, data-entry people, cleaners, and security guards. One of these security guards, a Samburu tribesman named Retunoi Lesiago, Kawango got a great kick out of telling me, had to sign his clinic contract with a thumb print. But in the intervening two years of employment, he'd learned to print his name.

The infrastructure Kawango had under her control was all to support a single venture, a clinical study that, after almost three years, had arrived at its halfway point. They were facing, she told me, two challenges: keeping track of the clients they'd already enrolled, 1,700 at this point, and recruiting 1,000 more young men they still needed to fulfill their mission. "We are doing pretty well on the first," she said. A major component of any clinical study is follow-up; in this case everybody they'd enrolled was supposed to return for regular medical check-ups, for HIV tests, and to provide the researchers with up-to-date lifestyle information. They were averaging about 90 percent, having, Kawango admitted, lost track of about 10 percent of their clients. But then she brightened—this was less than the 15 percent they had anticipated. From time to time, she said, they'd had to send trackers a full day's journey to Nairobi or Mombasa to find a client they needed to talk to, but the inconvenience did not seem to her extraordinary. "Most of our participants are jobless," she shrugged, "so we can't expect them to stay around; if they see an opportunity, they leave." On the second task of recruiting the thousand young men they still needed, she nodded toward the twenty-five sloping bodies outside her door aimlessly watching television while they waited for Martha or Millicent at the reception desk to send them on to a counsellor. One by one, Kawango believed, they would achieve their number.

On Monday morning, the other person mentioned by my taxi drivers, Bob Bailey, picked me up in the project van. Bailey, whom I'd first met two years earlier, was freshly returned from a visit back to Chicago and had brought his family, his wife and two sons, to Kisumu for a sabbatical year, settling them into a house not far from the Nyanza Club. That morning he had a problem to solve that was typical of his life here and a great deal different from the sorts of things he'd be doing had he remained in his classroom back in Illinois. A week earlier, a rainstorm and accompanying power surge had fried his laptop computer, and we needed to fetch it from the repair shop. The Indian-run shop was on the second floor of a dusty building that otherwise purveyed animal feed and over-stuffed furniture, the kinds of sofas that really dominate a room. We climbed the stairs to be greeted by the proprietor, a young man in a gleaming white shirt who shook hands with Bailey while proudly explaining that he had been able to save his files. He commenced opening various of them to demonstrate. "Oh god," exclaimed Bailey in mock horror. "Don't look at the pictures. They're all penises."

Bailey, an affable sort born in New York, started out his career not as a medical scientist but as an anthropologist. He earned his PhD (and published a *National Geographic* photo story) in 1989 studying pygmies in what was then Zaire. It would be a stretch, almost comic, to imagine the six-foot-two beanpole researcher mingling with four-foot-eight pygmies, but he got hooked on the African continent and, after obtaining a master's degree in epidemiology and public health, returned to Uganda and western Kenya to conduct surveys on attitudes and beliefs about male circumcision. Now he was co-researcher here with his Canadian counterpart, Stephen Moses.

With Bailey's once-again-functioning laptop under his arm, we climbed back into his vehicle to return to the clinic. Kawango greeted us by announcing that Ian Maclean had arrived and telling us to go straight to the lab to find him. In the lab we found him examining one of the refrigerators. The same power surge that damaged Bailey's laptop computer had disabled the refrigerator. But it was not going to be catastrophic, Maclean announced. The problem could be solved locally, and all he needed was to locate a new compressor. "Thank goodness, however, it wasn't the –80 degree fridge," he told us, "because for that we'd have to ship in a whole new one."

Through the lab door that morning new samples of blood serum, plasma, and urine arrived at a steady clip to be sorted by the Kenyan staff, Walter Otieno, Edith Nyagaya, and Lawrence Agunda. Surrounding them, along with the refrigerators, were tanks for shipping these specimens to the home labs for the researchers, eight time zones away. Back in Canada, Maclean, several times a year, organized a shipping container filled with whatever he thought the lab would need: rubber gloves, single-use scalpels, possibly a new refrigerator. The container would make its way from Winnipeg to Halifax by truck or train, then to Mombasa by sea, and then inland to Kisumu by truck. In the other direction, the blood serum, urine, and severed foreskins travelled by air. The amount of this specimen shipping was phenomenal. Maclean did the math for me: 2,700 clients times six visits to the clinic. Such a volume was actually more, the researchers determined, than their science needed; halfway into the project they had agreed they'd probably looked at enough foreskins back in Chicago to know everything they needed to know on that aspect of their study. Yet they could not stop sending them without first getting permission from both their funders and the various ethics boards that controlled their research.

All sorts of technologies were working to keep this project functioning. And the researchers had come to rely on them implicitly. Before the invention of e-mail, mused Bob Bailey, as he sat in front of his computer, everybody would have had to live on-site to do what the UNIM consortium were doing. Now he could easily stay in touch with Kawango from his office or house back in Chicago, transferring not only daily messages but also data. Stephen Moses, their other partner, was at that moment in India, but remained likewise in daily contact, again through e-mail. Later I found Maclean and Bailey huddled over the computer, examining another bit of novelty. On the screen Ian had called up an image purchased from a satellite photo service, a picture, blurry at first, that turned out on focussing to be an aerial photo of the town of Kisumu. Taken on an extraordinarily cloudless day, it showed the shores of Lake Victoria and the contours of the town. With Bailey now devotedly in thrall, he zoomed in all the way to individual houses, including the one where Bailey, his wife Nadine, and his two sons Alex and Nathan were staying for the duration of their sabbatical. "I didn't know my neighbour had a pool," Bailey exclaimed. To Maclean's mind, though, the aerial photo had larger possibilities, and Bailey was soon onside. The image scrolled to the poorer part of town, a scramble of tin roofs where there were no street names and no house numbers. "We could print out sections of this," he proposed, "and the recruiters could go in house to house while checking off on the map that they'd been there." Bailey agreed excitedly. Three years into their study, they had exhausted the bars and fishing docks around town and believed they needed now to go house to house to chase down their subjects. And they wanted to do it effectively and methodically. The technology of satellite imagery would help.

On Tuesday morning I was approached by one of the clinicians, Bernard Ayieko, who told me that if I wanted to watch a procedure I should come to the surgery in twenty minutes. I jumped at the opportunity with only the tiniest misgiving: it was a bit voyeuristic. But I convinced myself I'd never get another chance quite like this. The surgery was a smallish room just back of the waiting area and counsellors' offices. Ayieko, who was stocky, wore round, steel-framed glasses, and was thirty-nine years old, was already scrubbed and gowned as was his assistant, George Odhiambo. On the table, half under the green drape, lay a tall young man in his early twenties. Though he certainly looked the part when we'd sat down in his office earlier for a chat, Ayieko had stressed that he was not a real doctor. He had been trained as a clinician and had perfected his skill to do this specific surgery when posted with the Family Planning Association of Kenya and then, when he took the job at UNIM, had undergone, along with the two other surgeons, intensive additional training from a urologist flown in from America.

George handed me a mask and pointed to the corner where I had been designated to stand, out of the way though still assured of a good view. Through the window I could see burgundy-uniformed girls from the primary school next door well into their noisy recess. But back in the room it was an entirely different scene. Attempting friendliness, I offered my hello to the lanky young man stretched out on the table and asked him his name. Immediately Ayieko cautioned me, "because of the anonymity of the clinical trial you can only refer to him by his number." He would have to remain "Client 1665." Client 1665 grinned manically and rolled his eyes. His lower abdomen had been shaved though he had not yet been administered anaesthetic. "He is very nervous," conceded George, breaking the soft Swahili patter he had been maintaining in an effort to put the young man at ease. Ayieko readied his long needle. Client 1665 jumped. George continued to talk soothingly, much as he might to a high-strung racehorse.

Ayieko and George performed as many as three circumcisions a day, and by this point in the project's trajectory had done literally hundreds of the operations. Each took about ninety minutes from the beginning of prep, the scrubbing and laying out of the instruments, to the moment the patient finally got off the table and wobbled out the door. The actual operation itself took about forty minutes, though Ayieko, who liked to clock such things, said that the fastest they'd accomplished had been twenty-seven minutes. Usually the circumcision surgeries went smoothly, though not always. Three times, Ayieko confessed, his patients had bolted, right at the last moment when they were on the table, already shaved, and he himself was scrubbed, gloved, and gowned. "But that's okay," he said. "Some of them get scared, they're scared of the pain. So they have the right to leave."

Client 1665 might have been one of those who considered leaving, but instead remained fast, lying tense on the table, staring wide-eyed at the ceiling when he wasn't rolling his head to look over beseechingly at me. "Talk to me," he said at one point, "so that I don't have to think about what is going on down there." Before both of us knew it, though, the snip had been made. "Here," said George, holding the severed foreskin in his tweezers in front of the blinking young man's face. "Never to see it again." The suturing complete and bandages applied, Client 1665 gingerly slid off the table, worked himself carefully back into his jeans, and thanked us by weakly shaking hands all round. "You know," Ayieko cautioned him, "you're not to ride your bicycle for at least three days." The young man nodded and limped from the room. Outside the window, the burgundy uniformed schoolgirls were still at their play.

Bob Bailey first met Stephen Moses in 1996 at a meeting at the Centers for Disease Control in Atlanta, Georgia. It was a fated encounter in that the two men shared a niggling preoccupation. Moses, fifty-two years old, was born in Toronto, but had already lived for ten years, from the mid-1980s to 1996, in Nairobi where he had directed the collaboration's project to control AIDS and STDs in Kenya. Almost immediately after meeting Bailey, he started musing about an idea he'd been thinking about during all that time, the role of circumcision in HIV transmission. For his part, Bailey's ears perked up. Moses and Frank Plummer, at that time, had already published scientific papers pointing out that African men who had been circumcised suffered fewer STDs, including HIV infection. Plummer's research had also pointed out links between nasty STDs such as chancroid and gonorrhea and susceptibility to HIV, one of the theories being that the ulcers and sores that go with traditional STDs create portals for HIV entry. On top of this there were some as then untested theories about HIV receptor cells in foreskin tissue. To a man like Moses, with his public health bent, this was all he needed to be convinced. But what was missing was the definitive study, the clinical trial that would link circumcision and HIV prevention strongly enough to justify making circumcision part of the global anti-HIV strategy. And it would never happen, he lamented, unless a group could be brought together who would agree to be randomized, on the draw of a lottery consent to be circumcised—or not—and allow researchers to observe what transpired. Which is where an idea that would cement the collaboration emerged. Recalling the surveys he'd made not long before in western Kenya, Bailey piped up: "Maybe the Luo will."

Kenya is a country of more than 30 million people. But though it is a modern nation, it is also a tribal society. In the northwest corner, pressing up against Lake Victoria and the Ugandan border, 2 million strong, are the Luo. Of all the tribes in Kenya, the Luo fulfilled two conditions that made them appealing for such a study as the one Bailey and Moses wanted to carry out: they did not have a ritual of circumcision as part of their tradition and they had the country's highest HIV infection rate. When Bailey and Moses were making their proposal, the HIV rate in Kenya was widely accepted as 14 percent. In Luoland, however, it was more than twice that.

Bailey moved to Chicago and applied for funding to go to Kenya and Uganda to undertake "feasibility" studies. In these, basically, he would simply ask men and women in the Luo community and the group in Uganda that did not circumcise about their attitudes: would they consider accepting circumcision if it were offered? To his surprise, the majority said yes. General hygiene was one of the main reasons. If they were told there might be some medical benefit and it could be done safely, without too much pain, and it wasn't expensive, they were willing to be circumcised in spite of the cultural tradition. To make it even better, women supported the procedure for their husbands. Bailey then undertook a circumcision trial acceptability study. Gathering young men, he explained what would be involved in a clinical trial, then asked them what they would do. Would they volunteer to participate? Again, surprisingly, most of them said that they would. Moses and Bailey developed protocols, and applied for funding.

The politics of getting their study approved had in the end not been terribly difficult. Moses had his base in Nairobi while Bailey's anthropological surveys in Uganda and Kenya left him well-situated on the ground. He had gained the confidence of the provincial medical officer for the local Nyanza province and a force in Kenyan health care, Richard Muga. He'd been assured, as well, that Luo elders, while not having circumcision as part of their tradition, did not actively oppose it. With Muga's blessing, Bailey and Moses approached J.O. Ndinya-Achola, who was also a Luo, for an in-country partnership. Then they applied for grants to the NIH in the U.S. and the Canadian Medical Research Council (later to become Canadian Institutes of Health Research). The CIHR, in 2001, promised them $1.8 million CDN over five years; the NIH, $6 million US.

The subjects they decided on for the trial would be young men between eighteen and twenty-four years of age. This was a highly vulnerable as well as volatile group. Eighteen-year-old men in Kisumu had an HIV infection rate of 4 percent, which, by the time they reached twenty-four, spiked to 25 percent. Bailey and Moses had been told there were a potential 38,000 young men in the Kisumu district fitting into their demographic. They wanted 2,700 of them. To get into the study, each would have to test negative to HIV and be willing to be randomized—that is, agree to be circumcised right away if the lottery put him into that cohort or wait two years if he fell into the control group. Members of both groups had to agree to come back six times over a two-year period to continue to be tested and answer questions about their lifestyles and sexual habits. In return, they would receive some medical care and 300 KSh (about five dollars) for each visit to cover transportation expenses.

A couple of days after the session, in the surgery, Stephen Moses arrived from India, as did Allan Ronald, who had come to Kisumu from Canada via a few days in Uganda, and a young woman from Washington named Carolyn Williams, who watched over the clinical trial on behalf of the NIH. It was time to have a meeting, and everybody gathered round a table at the Nyanza Club. There were a number of issues on their plate. Bailey and Moses, who informally chaired the meeting, reiterated a persistent concern that they were somehow not yet getting a clientele that was fully typical of young Luo men. Bailey had been worried for some time that the HIV rate among those applying to be clients was too low. At about 10 percent, it was even lower than the Kisumu average. If they were to have any hope of showing that the procedure of circumcision was a protection, they would have to work with clients who were at high risk of contracting the virus. But where would they find them? To get a more "at-risk" group of people, they asked, should they be sending their recruiters into even rougher parts of town? Williams countered by reiterating the NIH's concerns about authenticity and credibility. She did not want the slightest whiff of coercion or enticement to creep into the study. She pointed out that she'd be quite happy if a certain percentage of potential clients dropped away before actually signing up since that would be evidence for her bosses back in Washington that the project maintained standards.

Down at the end of the table, Stephen Moses looked troubled. Something else, he said, had been nagging him for a long time, and that was what he called the Catch-22 of such a project. What if, he asked rhetorically, by simply being in the project the behaviour of the participants were to change? This, to him, would be highly problematic. "People might change their behaviour because of the counselling." Always ready with a joke, Bailey replied, "Yeah, if our counselling is effective, they'll all go home and start going to church." Ignoring him, Moses proceeded, deeply earnest: "My concern is that the incidence of HIV in the people in the trial won't be as high as in the general population," he said. "And the reason for that will be that people may change their behaviour because of the counselling. They may start doing what we're advising them to do, like wearing condoms. We have seen that in other trials."

His point underlined a true dilemma. The project may save lives, but the downside would be that such a response would render the scientific study useless. The researchers would not get the information they needed or could trust in order to come to definitive conclusions. For that to happen, everybody would have to behave exactly as they would have before the study, but how was that likely to be the case when they were surrounded in their visits to the clinic by posters warning of AIDS and offering safe-sex advice? The catch was that the clinic could neither morally nor ethically refrain from offering advice on safe sex and good health.

They batted this around for a while, then moved on. Allan Ronald brought up another matter, that of post-surgery problems, what the incidences were and how they were handling them. Under the rubric of adverse events, "AEs" in scientific jargon, the researchers were preoccupied with the need to find out and detail anything unhappy that followed the surgeries. "A 3 percent rate of some kind of infection is normal," Ronald pointed out. "But a big disaster would be if somebody should lose a penis." Everybody nodded. They didn't want that to happen.

Adverse events were a matter Bailey monitored closely. On the whole, he was satisfied. Ian Maclean observed that one of their clients had been shot by the police, "but that had nothing to do with his circumcision." Two percent was their targeted upper limit for incidents of adverse effects. Thus far, 2.5 percent had been the reality, though most had not been of a severe nature. The worst cases were things like stitches opening up before complete healing had taken place. One fellow, Bailey reported, had sex two times within eight days of his surgery, something he had been adamantly counselled against. Another rode his bicycle home after surgery, which did him no good. Poor hygiene had been a source of further complications, but nothing, he reported, seemed beyond manageable. Then there was more minutiae, such as the tensile strength of the sutures. "Let's face it," Ronald said, "if you're an eighteen- to twenty-year-old guy, you're going to have an erection every day, even the day after surgery." Everybody agreed that after three days the infection worry should be pretty much past, and after a week healing should be well progressed and the patients should be back riding their bicycles.

Finally they turned their attention to something Bailey had pronounced as an irritating bugbear: internal reviews. More visitors, also from Washington, were about to descend on them and the potential disruption lurked as a necessary inconvenience, but an inconvenience nonetheless, for the clinic and its staff. The visitors were called "monitors," and were coming to sift through all their paperwork. Under newly instituted regulations based on the system employed by drug trials back in North America, monitor teams were to visit each of the projects under NIH jurisdiction, including theirs, twice a year. All documents had to be made available so that the monitors could take a fine-tooth comb to them. The concerns prompting the program, Bailey agreed, were legitimate: to check that subjects of studies were properly informed and protected. But he looked as glum as he would were he facing an income tax audit. "It has radically changed the whole business of research," he lamented. "Five years ago there was nothing of this." He considered it a layer of irritating extra work and also questioned its effect. Did the system, he asked, really increase protection of the subjects? The monitors would look at documents, but not interview the staff or the clients. "The fact that you have a piece of paper," Bailey asked, "what does that mean? Does it guarantee that the subject understands?"

These sorts of questions were of acute interest to the scientists as well, especially to Bailey, whose main hat, the one he could not seem to get rid of no matter how deeply he got enmeshed in medical science, was that of the anthropologist. There was more to medical research, he readily averred, than simply testing medical procedures; the whole life and history of a society or community was wrapped up in beliefs and practices that impinged on how the research that called itself "science" would be viewed, accepted, cooperated with, and carried out.

A good example of the conundrum they faced might have become evident had they been able to get inside the head of somebody like Client 1665. It would have been quite a journey to know everything that was going on for Client 1665, both at the moment of his surgery and also in the days leading up to his submitting himself for it. What had really motivated him? What had convinced him that this was something he should look into and volunteer for? Was he moved by self-interest? Was the promise of perpetual health care and the prospect of pocket change every time he came to the clinic all it took to make him do it? Was he persuaded personally by the possibility that circumcision might be a form of prevention that could save his life (though all counselling given the clients stressed the point that the jury was still out, only their study might prove something)? Or was he moved in some altruistic way by the larger argument put forward by the foreign researchers and their local staff about this being some vital experiment in the war against AIDS? Was there something in him that made him want to be part of something larger than his own life? Whatever his motivating reasons, he had, after all, undergone an excruciating surgery, one that would take him out of commission in both work and play for not some small amount of time. He had submitted to an altering of his natural body in a way that was neither popularly accepted nor even recommended by the culture within which he had grown up and lived. And he had done so simply on the say-so of two doctors from America. In their eyes he had become a foot soldier in the war against AIDS. But was that how he saw himself? And was that how his community would see him?

From Bailey's standpoint a study such as theirs necessitated an interaction with the community as a whole and included matters from public relations to intelligence gathering. One day he introduced me to a young man, Dipesh Pabari. Born in Kisumu, Pabari was a fourth-generation Asian (Indian) Kenyan with a master's degree in anthropology from the University of London's School of Oriental and African Studies. He was twenty-six years old, and in twenty years would look like the actor Ben Kingsley. Desiring to learn as much as they could about what the people of Kisumu thought of them and what they were doing, Bailey and Moses had hired Pabari to look at perceptions held by people in the community at large. The assignment was not only to accumulate and collate a record of those perceptions, but also to try to discern how those might have been formed and how they were influenced by culture, both that of the local community and the traditional culture of the Luo. It was anthropology, psychology, and cultural studies rolled into one, and a project Pabari relished. When I finally sat down with him, the young man told me he was euphoric about his task. "I'm being paid to get to know my community," he said. He was accomplishing his mission by getting on his bicycle every morning and scooting around Kisumu's bars and markets in order to talk and to listen.

From Pabari I learned the difference between a "whistle," in the jargon of young Kisumu men, an uncircumcised penis, and a "spear," one that is circumcised. He also explained something that he said had surprised the researchers. Circumcision was becoming increasingly common among all the tribes in Kenya, and by not being circumcised the Luo were in fact a bit on the outs— something that did not sit well with the young. Among these young there was developing, Pabari discerned, a strong desire to conform, to act and look like Kenya's other tribes. Even young Luo women were reportedly coming to prefer men with "spears." For Bailey and Moses, this information allayed one of their great fears, that they would have a problem recruiting. Initially Pabari said he encountered some negative opinion about the project, not to mention some weird rumours. A few people told him that circumcision was a form of devil worship, while others passed on hearsay that the clinic was collecting foreskins, drying them, and sending them to America to be made into handbags. But negative views turned out to be the exception. "Ninety-nine percent of the reaction," he insisted, "is favourable."

He faced one myth, however, that was broadly enough held it ought, he said, to cause worry. With sufficient frequency to make him take note, he came upon people who told him they believed getting tested was not simply how one found out one had AIDS, it was in fact the way one *caught* AIDS. "My cousin, my friend, my colleague," they would tell him, "went and got tested and now he has AIDS." The implication in their minds seemed to be that if he had not gone to the clinic for that test he would still be fine. As a form of denial from uneducated people who dreaded bad news, this was perhaps understandable. But such a view still held colossal consequences. Immediately, for the research project, it could cancel out the good news on the recruiting front. The first thing required for one to enroll in the study was an HIV test, and such an attitude could keep people away, especially those at the low end of society, the higher-risk groups the scientists needed. In the broader picture, such a myth fed by such misinformation could prove disastrous in battling an epidemic like AIDS.

On the issue of whether or not circumcising was okay, Pabari's finding that the project was not transgressing some deeply held community belief caused Bailey and Moses to heave a sigh of relief. Opinions pro and con with regard to circumcision and its importance in relation to the cornerstones of Luo culture, in fact, appeared to be neutral in general and leaning toward positive among the young. A deeper understanding was offered, back at the clinic, by Maurice Onyango, one of the counsellors assigned to deal with clients when they first came through the door. Onyango was a proud Luo and confirmed that the tribe did have traditions that set it apart. But those were changing. A soft-spoken fellow in a green-striped golf shirt, he personified the transition through which his tribe (indeed, much of Kenyan society) was passing at the beginning of the twenty-first century. He explained that his father had three wives and that two siblings, the children of one of those wives, had gone through a traditional Luo coming-of-age rite called "Nago," which involved removing the bottom four incisor teeth. But Onyango had all his teeth and only one wife. And while Luo tradition was not to circumcise, the taboo against it, he confirmed, agreeing with what Pabari had been finding, was not strong. Young men were embracing it, he believed, especially when they were told about hygiene and when they learned about the possibility of lower susceptibility to sexually transmitted diseases.

Since Nago was no longer widely practised, Onyango said Luo boys were left without any real initiation ceremony. Which was a matter that appeared to be fine with him. When Kenya's largest tribe, the Kikuyu, for example, had a ceremony for circumcision, "there is," he said, "a lot of pain." When it came to getting circumcised, in Onyango's opinion, "most people prefer the hospital method." Onyango pointed to a room where the follow-up questionnaires were kept. The system of documentation at the project was extensive and boxes of questionnaires waiting for dissemination were stacked to the ceiling. He pulled one and opened it. Clients on their second follow-up visit after surgery were to answer the following questions:

Are you satisfied or dissatisfied with the results of the circumcision?

If you have had sexual intercourse since your circumcision, did your sex partner express any opinion about your circumcision?

If yes, was your partner
    1: very satisfied
    2: somewhat satisfied
    3: somewhat dissatisfied
    4: very dissatisfied

Out in the clinic waiting room eight or ten strapping young men lounged on the couches, eyeing a religious revival program on the TV until Rosemary, behind the reception desk, switched the channel to cartoons. The sprawling young men—like Client 1665—were more clients or would-be clients waiting for their interviews. Among them sat a smiley-looking chap with dreadlocks who came over to introduce himself, informing me that he was not one of the clients, but a worker. He motioned me to follow him outside, where—after a gentle hand-shake I was becoming accustomed to among these fellows, limp and completely unaggressive, like a tentative gift—he shyly began to tell his story. Ten years earlier, when he was fifteen, Alex—or Rasta-man as he had come to be called because of the dreadlocks—had drifted from a village in the countryside into Kisumu where his lack of job and money immediately relegated him to living on the street, essentially homeless. "To survive, I scavenged at the dump, I lived in a hand-made shanty," he said. But then he had been recruited by the foreign scientists and now his job was to gather in to the project as many as possible of those same street people who still lived hand to mouth. Some of them were part-time fishermen, some were *boda-boda* drivers. Some got by, as had Alex, scavenging at the dump. These were the kinds of young men Bailey and Moses liked to sign up because they saw them as being at higher risk than young men from the more settled elements of society. As such they would stand to benefit more if the project's hypothesis turned out to be true, and, more important for science, because of their casual lifestyle they offered a higher probability of putting the hypothesis to a real test.

Once these young men walked through the door of the clinic, however, they were no longer in the world they understood or that operated by their rules. They entered a system that was not African by construction but North American. The clinical trial was an internationally proscribed world with, like a chess game, its own rules. And these rules were stringent. If they were not followed, the results of entire years of work could be termed suspect or thrown out altogether. The list of things around which there was little compromise was a long one, and it seemed to trouble Alex greatly. What it did serve to highlight were the incongruities between the North American way of looking at and doing things and the African way. On every fine North American point, Alex's Kenyan view, and especially his view as a person from the street, diverged. The foreign overseers and monitors would lecture him, along with the rest of the staff, about their rules and protocols. But he, as often as not, could only quietly consider those to be absurd. For example, the clients were promised health care for two years and to receive payment each time they visited the clinic. For the North Americans running and overseeing and monitoring and ultimately judging the project, it was important that it never appear that such an exchange was persuasive or in-fluential. In the eyes of scientific officials, especially those back in North America, participants in the trial always had to be seen as having come to it out of their own free will, uninfluenced by extraneous considerations. But the street-level perspective of Rasta-man begged to differ. And in that was wrapped up more of the conundrums of long-distance research in developing countries: the poverty of the participants was immensely relevant to their having made the decision to join the study, to have come along with him to enrol and participate. "The offer of free health care is truly significant," he pronounced firmly, "because otherwise they cannot afford medicine. Perhaps it is the decisive motivation." As well, the 300 KSh one was set to receive in return for each visit was significant because if you were a *boda-boda* driver you would have to peddle all the way across town with a fare loaded behind you on your bicycle to get only 10 percent of that.

Rasta-man nonetheless confirmed part of the information delivered already by Pabari and Onyango: young men were impatient to get circumcised. They were actively seeking out the clinic to obtain an operation that, in his view, many could not otherwise afford. A circumcision at a commercial clinic would cost thirty to sixty dollars, or a hundred fares for a *boda-boda* driver.

As it happened, when the monitors visited, they did unearth something they considered an irregularity: a piece of paper that was part of the protocol between the researchers and their subjects and needed to be put on record with all the partnering institutions either had not been filed in the offices of the University of Nairobi, or had been lost there. The matter, according to regulations, fell under the category "breach of ethics" and prompted the monitors to pronounce that until things got sorted out UNIM would be obliged to close its doors. The scientists were dismayed, mostly because they knew what would ensue would be a bureaucratic circus, a lengthy rigmarole of documents and explanations sent endlessly on the rounds from Nairobi to Winnipeg to Washington to Chicago, institution to institution to institution, desk to desk to desk. It was all exhausting and upsetting. "I didn't sleep for nine months," Bailey later admitted.

The issue was raised by the U.S.-based member of the monitoring team who questioned whether the researchers had proper clearance for some of the substudies they were undertaking. When the matter arrived in front of the chair of the ethics board at the University of Nairobi, he became worried about what was going on way off in Kisumu and decided to take the safest course of action. An independent team was dispatched to go through all of UNIM's paperwork. Because they were dealing with a high-profile clinical trial, the ethics committee did not want it to seem as if they were being railroaded into blanket approvals, especially when it was an American who had drawn the matter to their attention. Ultimately, it was determined that everything was fine, though UNIM changed their consent forms to make them more explicit. In Moses's view, that was all fair enough, "but the problem was that it took a very long time for them to do their investigation, lots of paper flew back and forth, just dragged on while they continued reviewing." The episode put the project on hold for several months, during which time they did no procedures or recruiting. According to both Bailey and Moses, "it cost us time and money."

CHAPTER NINE

Legitimizing Circumcision

In July 2005, a front-page story in the *Wall Street Journal* reported that an African circumcision trial had been halted. Robert Bailey and Stephen Moses were not the only scientists pursuing the question of male circumcision and its possible impact on HIV. In South Africa a similar study had been underway, conducted by a French researcher from the Université de Paris.[1] Bertrand Auvert, with his South African colleague Dirk Taljaard, had enrolled 3,000 young men age eighteen to twenty-four in order to circumcise half of them and, like Bailey and Moses, keep track of the results. In March 2005, nine months before their study was scheduled to come to its end, their data and safety monitoring board (DSMB), an independent scientific review body to which all scientists undertaking studies need to report, ordered Auvert and Taljaard to stop their work. A preliminary unlocking of their data showed the discrepancy in HIV infections between their two cohorts to be an astonishing 65 percent. In other words, male circumcision, at least in their group, was cutting HIV infection by upwards of two-thirds. "It would not be moral," declared the DSMB, "in the light of such astounding data, to continue with a group from who you were withholding the possibility of becoming circumcised." The study, it would seem, had proved its point; instead of waiting out their term, these young men should be free to get circumcised immediately if they so wished.

Bailey and Moses, naturally, were anxious to know what this development would mean for them and their study. They were not so far along as the South Africans had been, yet might their data safety monitoring board follow suit and agree that continued trial was not only a waste of time but unethical with respect to their control group? They were quickly reassured that would not be the case. The DSMB that had looked at their up-to-the-minute results recommended the

Kisumu trial continue. "Obviously," Moses recounted, "they must have felt that there was not a strong enough difference in HIV rates between circumcised and uncircumcised men to stop the trial. This may be because we have not yet had enough follow-up to be able to conclude that there is a real statistical difference, or there may not be one. We don't know."

What the decision that they should continue meant as well, it seemed on the face of it, was a recognition that somewhere a clinical trial needed to go all the way through to its conclusion. If mass circumcision of African men was going to become a strategy in the battle against AIDS, one had to think that should not come about based on a hypothesis and trials that pointed in the right direction but then got aborted. There should be at least one and perhaps more than one completed trial in order for there to be anything near scientific certainty.

What Bailey and Moses did know was that about forty of their subjects had become infected with HIV. But since they were still "blinded" (which is to say, forbidden by the random trial to identify their subjects, though their monitoring board was not), they did not know which group these men were in, or, if they were from both, what the balance was. For his part, Bailey found the forty sero-conversions encouraging in that it was a number that was in the range of what they had expected. "We predicted a sero-conversion rate of about 1 percent among the circumcised men and 2.5 percent among the non-circumcised group," he said. "Since 40 turns out to be 1.7 percent, or halfway between our two numbers, we can assume that we are right where we thought we would be." What these numbers also did was reassure them that the issue of behavioural change they had worried about was at least not yet affecting their numbers.

In June of 2006, the UNIM project's clinical trial landed again in front of the data and safety monitoring board. Again, Bailey and Moses sat on pins and needles waiting for the board's decision. Again, their project was spared, but only provisionally. They were told they would be looked at once more in another six months. When this happened, on December 12, 2006, at least a year in advance of their scheduled completion, their research project was at last halted. As the monitors had pronounced eighteen months earlier with the South African research, their numbers were turning out to be so good it would be unethical to the young men in the control group to hold them back any longer from seeking circumcision if they so wanted. Without completing a full clinical trial, those championing circumcision had, by a two-to-one margin, proved their point. With additional authors Kawango Agot, Carolyn Williams, Ian Maclean, and J.O. Ndinya-Achola, Bailey and Moses published the results of their study, as far as it had gone, in the *Lancet*.[2] Looking at 2,784 young men in Luoland, they reported the two-year incidence of HIV among the half of them that got circumcised was 2.1 percent; among the control group, the half who had not been circumcised, 4.2 percent. The reduction in the risk of acquiring HIV was 53 percent. It was one of the few bits of good news on the HIV front that year.

The interesting detail about male circumcision as a strategy for HIV/AIDS prevention is the story of how long it took and the stubborn hurdle-filled journey to get the procedure and its effects accepted by the big thinkers and the big agencies in the global AIDS business. The first evidence—mostly from the Manitobans—came available in the 1980s, close to the epidemic's outbreak. Yet it was not until 2000 that the first trials were organized, and comprehensive circumcision as an HIV prevention strategy only got rolled out ten years after that.[3]

Very early, in 1986 and 1987, attention to the possible role circumcision might play came when Frank Plummer was studying men attending the Casino Clinic in Nairobi, just after HIV came on the scene. He and his colleagues were exploring associations between HIV and other STDs, especially genital ulcers. Stephen Moses reports on the process: "For some reason they decided to ask people about circumcision, I guess because circumcision had been shown in the past to have associations with various other STDs. We really weren't expecting to find much, it was just kind of routine background question. It doesn't hurt to ask." As Plummer looked at the data, it seemed that those men who had been circumcised showed a remarkably reduced risk of acquiring HIV. This surprised him to such an extent he summoned Allan Ronald, chief of medicine at the University of Manitoba, to tell him, "believe it or not, the strong association was there." That, claims Moses, was really the first time it was noted. "A couple of others had speculated but with no evidence. The data from Frank, working with trainee Bill Cameron, was the first solid clinical data that there might be something to it."[4]

In 1989, an American team led by John Bongaarts of the Population Council published a paper showing a correspondence between sub-Saharan regions where men traditionally were not circumcised and higher HIV rates.[5] Moses himself, based on analysis done in Kenya, came to the same conclusion, publishing his findings in the *International Journal of Epidemiology* a year later.[6] But not much happened, prompting the medical journalists to weigh in. In 1996, in an article in *Scientific American*, John and Pat Caldwell wrote, "Surprisingly, the publication of these two papers did not excite much interest. The WHO's Global Program on AIDS emphasized that Moses and his team could not point to any physiological mechanism to explain how lack of circumcision was implicated in an increased risk of HIV infection; the research simply demonstrated a statistical correlation between circumcision, chancroid or syphilis, and HIV infection. Consequently, other researchers gave the finding little weight."[7]

The Caldwells were on a lengthy quest to get an epidemiological handle on what was happening in Africa. They went against the conventional wisdom of organizations like the WHO, by pressing forward conclusions that "the link between circumcision and elevated levels of HIV infection appears robust." This was the case particularly in concert with customs of multiple sex partners and other unsafe sexual practices. "In the AIDS belt," they wrote, "lack of male circumcision in combination with risky sexual behaviour such as having multiple sex partners, engaging in sex with prostitutes and leaving chancroid untreated, has led to rampant HIV transmission."[8]

While the research camp pushed, those who directed health care delivery were decidedly more cautious, even resistant. Stephen Moses went to meetings of the WHO in Geneva only to encounter what he felt was a brick wall. Opinion in the West, pre-dating HIV/AIDS, had long been against circumcision, holding that while a rite honoured by certain religious groups (both Jews and Muslims, as well as numerous African tribes), it was outside of that something of the past not the future, a meaningless mutilation, even kind-of primitive, and not worth considering in the context of modern health. This became even more the case when publicity campaigns about female genital mutilation in backward corners of the globe got ethicists up in arms. Horror stories from that front provoked the public and the media to easily lump the two together, female mutilation and male circumcision, with little effort at making a distinction. When AIDS came along, according to Moses, circumcision seemed like it might be important, but it was also controversial. A lot of groups within the AIDS world were vehemently opposed to considering circumcision, especially the Europeans, who had grown skeptical about circumcision mostly for cultural reasons. "They did not even wish to revive the discussion and open up consideration on an abstract level," he said. Some seemed to fear as well that giving the practice the imprimatur of medical sanction might in turn lead to ethnic hostilities in places where tribal customs and traditions differed.

The policy agencies, for their part, admitted later that they were slow to properly consider circumcision as a prevention strategy for AIDS, but they believe also that their caution was justified. Gary Slutkin, an American from Chicago who worked between 1987 and 1994 for the WHO Global Program on AIDS says, "the main things for the WHO to recommend a policy are proven effectiveness and feasibility. If you have a strategy to use against a disease or an epidemic, it has to be one that can actually be rolled out."[9] He says this regularly placed the WHO between researchers on the one side, eager to try things, and the real, practical world on the other. "In the middle, WHO always had to try to be the honest broker." Slutkin recounts that in 1990 the agency commissioned a worldwide review of what strategies might work against HIV/AIDS, scanning the globe and polling experts in the scientific community. While circumcision was mentioned in the returns, he points out that there had been at that time "no firm studies" of effective intervention. Under the other mantra of WHO, "do no harm," it would not have been responsible, in his opinion, to go out and "start snipping young men." Slutkin recalls raising the matter with two African epidemiologist colleagues, a Ghanaian and a Zambian, and their response was that circumcision was not only unproven but likely unfeasible. "They were in our research units and both told me they felt male circumcision was a 'no starter,' Africans would not go for it," says Slutkin. In the end, though, he adds, "Bob [Bailey] and Steve [Moses] proved something that should have been proved earlier."

By the late 1990s, the ground on the validity of circumcision began to shift ever so slightly. The "policy" organizations—WHO and UNAIDS—began using more accommodating language, saying things like "the evidence is suggestive," but emphasizing that they could not develop policy without the evidence of a clinical trial. Stephen Moses says that Plummer "would argue that people took far too long, but the potential complications of the surgery were an issue, plus the other problem, behavioural inhibition. Circumcision isn't a 100 percent protection from HIV, but what if people started acting like it was, adopting more risky sexual behaviour?"

The possibility of behavioural change had all along been a bugbear, something Stephen Moses thought about while the clinical trial was going on, and something that will always be a feature of concerns about the strategy of circumcision. It may be a 60 percent protection, but 60 percent is not 100 percent. During the clinical trial, his concerns had to do with scientific authenticity. Given the potential that sizable numbers of the participants might start behaving differently after entering it, could any trial be authentic, he wondered? Could truly reliable information emerge when other variables had been thrown into the mix, when the young men had been counselled into safe-sex practices as part of their participation? When the South African results were the first to become public, he paused to worry: what if the lower HIV rates among those subjects were in fact a result of changes in behaviour and not a result of circumcision at all?

In an attempt to shed some light on the degree to which this might be a factor, he and Bailey, about two-thirds of the way along in their trial, decided to undertake another study. Bailey got one of his graduate students from the University of Illinois to engineer what they called a "disinhibition" study. The student was to try to collect hard data about the actual behaviour of young men and construct that against the information the trial's follow-up was gathering.[10] To get it going they procured a little house across the road from the clinic in which they installed two young Kenyans, Evans Otieno and Nicholas Okul, with instructions to interview as many of the young men coming and going from the clinic as possible and try to get answers to the sticky question of whether either participation in the project or a circumcision had altered how they behaved sexually. There were two sides to the question of what implications their behaviours might have for the young men's HIV vulnerability. Whereas Stephen Moses worried about too many of them behaving more carefully, there also emerged a concern that they behave *less* carefully under the illusion that seemed to persist on the street, that being circumcised provided "full" protection against HIV. Otieno and Okul, in their interviews, were to try to determine how successfully the message that this is *not* the case got implanted. When I paid a visit they were still some distance from completing their study and coming up with their academic report, but Nicholas Okul confided that, given the volume of information and advice available to the young men concerning HIV and the importance of safe-sex practices, depressingly little seemed to have been sinking in. Or at least behaviour had not aligned itself with knowledge. Young men had been seated in rooms surrounded by posters proclaiming the dangers of AIDS and given information about condoms. They had been instructed carefully that the jury was still out on the protective capacity of a circumcision and how, even at best, it would be but a partial protection. Yet, in spite of it all, a good number confessed to Okul and Otieno that the sex they were now having was casual and undertaken with no more care than it had ever been. To explain this, Nicholas slipped into religious analogy, referring to those who were recalcitrant as "backsliders." "Talking about AIDS," he said, continuing the religious metaphor, "is like preaching the gospel. You may preach every day, but how many are saved?"

The Kisumu clinical trial closed in 2006. Once results were announced, a large press conference was organized at the headquarters of the NIH in Washington, D.C. Stephen Moses, by then into a new project in India, was patched in by a cell phone teleconference. He was delighted to be part of it, even though the event got started at 2 a.m. local Indian time. Various heavy hitters were at the other end, including Anthony Fauci of the NIH and Kevin de Cock, head of HIV programs at the WHO. The triumph of the new information moved impressively forward. In April 2007, the previously cautious WHO convened a major consultation in Montreux, Switzerland, bringing together all stakeholders—government, UN, academics—fifty people in total. This meeting proved a complete turnaround from what had been the case previously. The majority opinion was that the data was now compelling, and it was important to ratchet up circumcision, especially in certain situations such as countries where HIV prevalence was high and men were not traditionally circumcised. The WHO promptly developed protocols that mandated use of a local anaesthetic and that there be parental consent for minors up to age seventeen. Meanwhile, the Kenyan government put out an official policy on circumcision.

Three years later, by 2010, the UNIM clinic in Kisumu had been transformed into a full-time centre for circumcision provision. Kawango Agot, the U.S.-trained local Kisumu native remained in charge of a PEPFAR-funded program to ramp up male circumcision. All levels of officialdom and society had come on board. The government of Kenya had set a goal of 100,000 circumcisions a year. The potential was great: in Nyanza province alone, the potential clientele numbered 600,000, against which resources in Kisumu estimated they could deliver 30,000 to 40,000 per year. All manner of people were seeking out UNIM; parents were bringing their ten year-old boys to the clinic for a circumcision. Agot and her colleagues organized training teams that then helped produce 700 case workers. The UNIM clinic was an in-town service; in the surrounding countryside and villages, mobile teams would each perform a dozen circumcisions a day. By the end of 2009, 90,136 circumcisions had been performed in Nyanza Province.

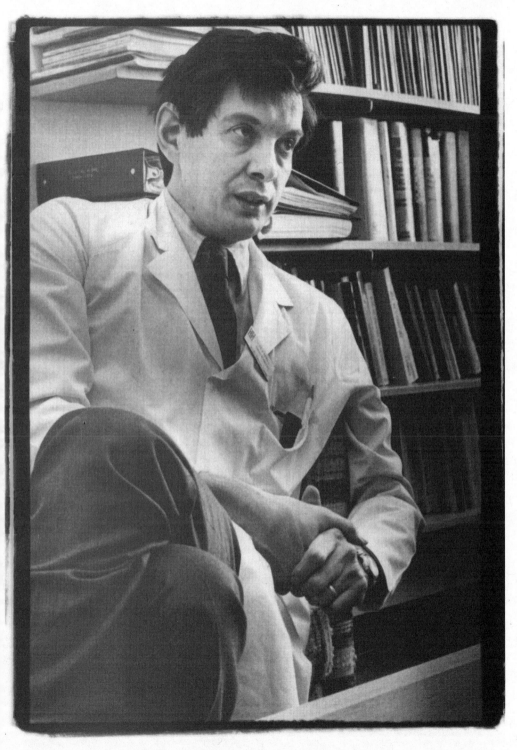

Allan Ronald in Winnipeg, 1978, soon after leading an effort to combat a chancroid outbreak in the city. UNIVERSITY OF MANITOBA ARCHIVES AND SPECIAL COLLECTIONS.

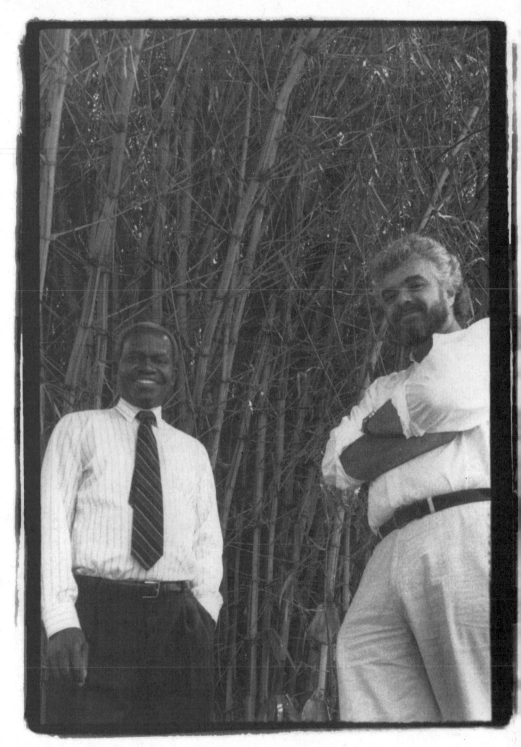

J.O. Ndinya-Achola and Frank Plummer at the University of Nairobi, 1994.
PHOTO BY CHERYL ALBUQUERQUE.

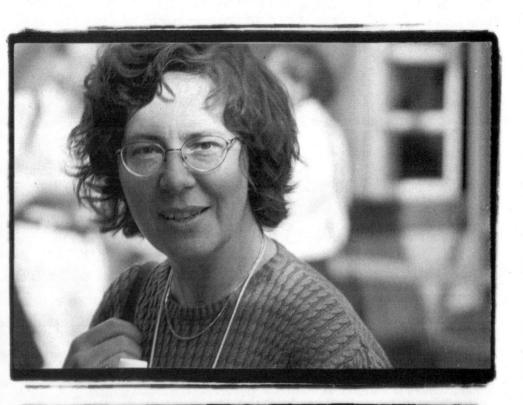

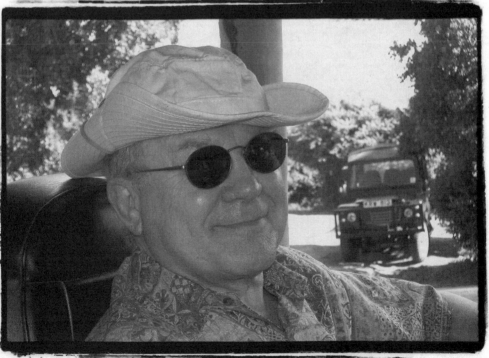

Joan Kreiss and King Holmes of the University of Washington. PHOTOS BY RUPERT KAUL AND COURTESY UNIVERSITY OF WASHINGTON.

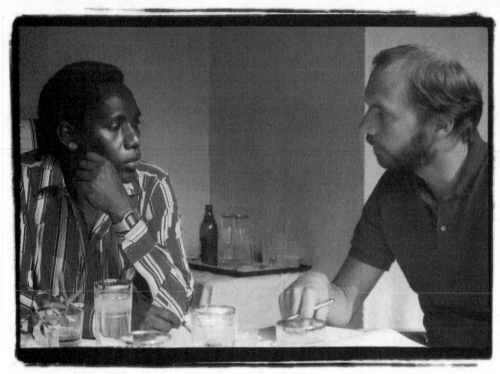

Herbert Nsanze and Peter Piot, early 1980s. PHOTO COURTESY PETER PIOT.

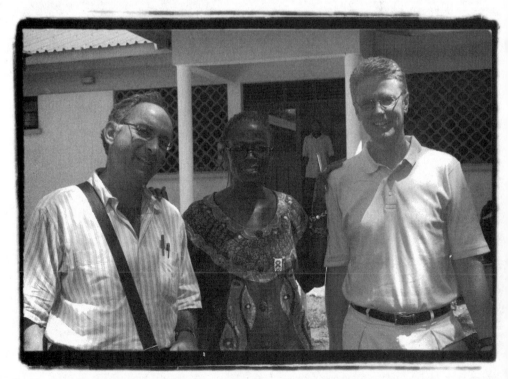

Stephen Moses, Kawango Agot, and Robert Bailey outside the UNIM Clinic in Kisumu, Kenya, 2002. PHOTO BY LARRY KROTZ.

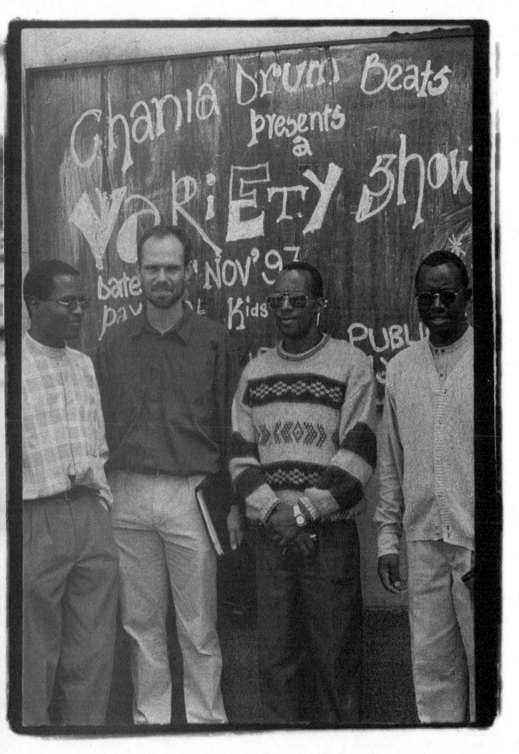

Ephantus Njagi, Rupert Kaul, Mwangi Kimani (Joshua's brother), and Joshua Kimani.
PHOTO COURTESY RUPERT KAUL.

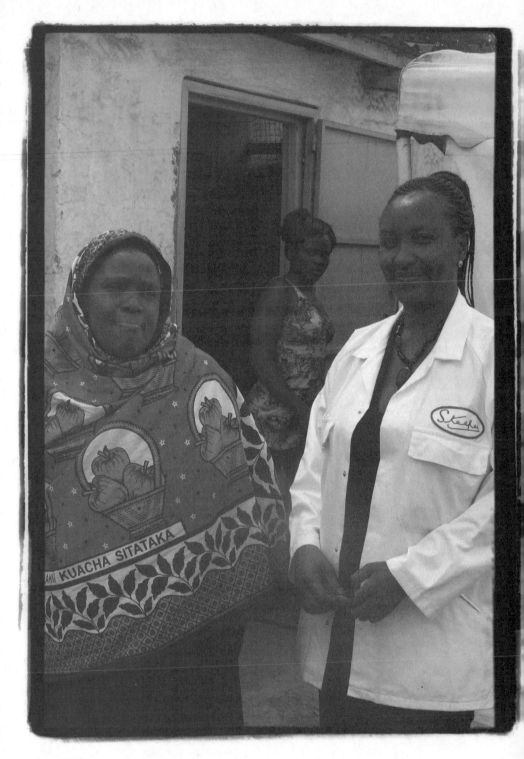

Hawa Chelangat, one of Nairobi's "persistent sero-negative" sex workers, with nurse Jane Kamene, 2010. PHOTO BY LARRY KROTZ.

CHAPTER TEN

Unfinished Business

O n a Friday afternoon in January 2007, a group of dignitaries, including the Canadian minister of health, gathered under the hot sun on the grounds of the University of Nairobi medical school to cut a ribbon and open a brand new building. If buildings can be iconic and symbolic, this one surely was. Rising at the end of the breezeways of the medical school campus, this was a handsome four-story structure with one glass wall, and the others plastered in rose-coloured stucco. It included floors of offices and a research laboratory capable of handling the most hazardous of pathogens. The new building represented the manner in which, after almost thirty years, the collaboration among the universities and researchers would continue, and, as a gift from Canada, it acknowledged both the growing needs and the growing capabilities of Kenya and East Africa. It was going to be a lot of things: home to one of only three such high-level labs in all of Africa (Johannesburg, in South Africa, has a Level 4 lab, and Gabon has one designated as Level 3), and home as well to an Institute for Tropical and Infectious Diseases, unique to Africa and modelled on the best such institutes in Europe and North America. To celebrate it, a lot was on the line—for everybody. The Canadians, along with the minister of health, Tony Clement, were represented by Emőke Szathmáry, the woman who had been University of Manitoba president through some of the most challenging years of the relationship. Frank Plummer had returned to Kenya for the first time after an absence of almost seven years. On the Kenyan side, when word went round that their minister of health, Charity Kaluki Ngilu, might not attend due to illness, a visibly irritated university vice-chancellor, George Magoha, promptly got on the phone. Soon, Ngilu's car drove up.

The gathered dignitaries entered, with everybody else, into a high-octane celebration: choirs sang, students from the university English department recited a poem they had composed, titled in Kikuyu, "Ta Imagini" (Just Imagine). Its second verse went:

> Ta imagini
> That all the scientists stood hand in hand
> Marched side by side
> Forming one mighty research foundation
> Sweeping all human diseases
> And rolling them into the ocean
> Ta imagini

A young man, who at the International AIDS Conference in Toronto a year earlier had been presented by Canada's minister of health with a video camera so he could record the story of HIV/AIDS in his Kenyan community, showed up to be reunited with Tony Clement. The Canadian minister, standing shoulder to shoulder with the other dignitaries, tried to frame the moment in a grand, transnational manner. "The best response to perils that don't respect borders," Clement told the assembled guests, "is ensuring that our knowledge and action also transcends geographic boundaries." When he got to his speech, Magoha used it to chastise his government for its practice of continuing to exact import duties on items, such as the equipment for the new lab, that were meant for the good of Kenya. Clement and Ngilu then planted trees on the lawn in front of the new structure.

A substantial aspect of both the new building and the legacy the collaboration was trying to create, was the infectious diseases laboratory that occupied parts of two of its floors. A Level 3 lab like this one is designed with sufficient bio-hazard security features that, beyond HIV, it can secure such dastardly viruses as Marburg, Ebola, and Rift Valley fever, none of which are strangers to central Africa. In 1967, an outbreak of Ebola had killed 318 people in what was then Zaire; in 2004, Marburg killed 227 in Angola. The fatality rates, should either appear again and get out of control, are in the 90 percent range. The laboratory, outfitted in shiny, sterile stainless steel, what one would expect of a highly secure laboratory, would stand like a centurion, ready to do its protective part.

What distinguishes a Level 3 designation starts in its very design. In a Level 2 lab the individual laboratory technician is protected by working under a safety cabinet, a hood not unlike a kitchen fan, which sucks all air particles into a vent and carries them away. Level 3 labs, which house more dangerous pathogens, are equipped with systems that direct air flow away not just from an individual bench, but from the entire room, removing it from the work being done and sending it out through filters fine enough to remove even the tiniest infectious agents. No street clothes are permitted in these labs, the technicians are gowned, and eye protection is mandatory. All surfaces are designed to be easily decontaminated. The stainless steel benches for this new lab were provided by the University of Manitoba who bought them as surplus from Canada's National Microbiology Laboratory in Winnipeg and had them shipped to Africa.

Overseeing a lab with such high safety standards and such demanding possibilities made its director, David Mburu, puff up with pride. Mburu, who came over from the animal lab of the government of Kenya, was hired in 2006. His first task was to wait impatiently for his new lab's completion and then, sitting in his small office beneath photos of the dignitaries at the building's opening ceremonies, he needed to wait for the research grants to begin flowing so he could put technicians to work behind those shiny stainless-steel benches. "Like a fire department," he told me, "you can't handle a real fire if you haven't been practising." He hoped not to have to confront any real-life deadly agents, Ebolas and Marburgs, until his staff had been busy with regular projects designed to keep them sharp.

Bringing in those research grants will depend increasingly on what happens in the offices on the floor above Mburu. Behind the door announcing the "Institute of Tropical and Infectious Diseases," sat its director, another Kenyan, Benson Estambale. The dream for an institute like this went all the way back to the mid-1990s. The work of the international universities in the Nairobi collaboration had grown to be so extensive and complex that it was believed they should be handled by something larger than the departments of microbiology of the various schools, as had been the case until then. When Frank Plummer put together a proposal for an institute, he had in mind those in Europe, in London and Liverpool, Copenhagen and Ghent, centres of expertise on infectious diseases particular to the tropical parts of the world. Alas, there were no funds to see such a dream through, and the idea was shelved. But only temporarily. In Manitoba, the proposal was used persistently and quietly to troll for money, and in 1999, after almost a decade, officials there got back to the vice-chancellor of the University of Nairobi, George Magoha, with an offer. If the University of Manitoba were to find funds for a building, would Nairobi find the required real estate and put an administration in place? This was coincidental to the time Plummer was leaving Kenya to take up residence back in Winnipeg and an eventual new job as director of the National Microbiology Laboratory. At his urging, the University of Manitoba put together a proposal to present to the Canada Foundation for Innovation's first international competition that had let it be known it was ready to look at projects that had a strong Canadian dimension but a position outside the boundaries of Canada. If it were to become a reality, the proposed institute would be owned in partnership by the universities of Nairobi and Manitoba and would have its own board of directors. To everyone's happy satisfaction, the proposal did succeed; the Manitobans persuaded the CFI that Nairobi should be the location for their first venture outside Canada to make links in world infectious diseases control. The requisite follow-up moved with lightning-speed. Approvals flew through the university senate and other supervisory councils in Nairobi, and in 2003 George Magoha and J.O. Ndinya-Achola journeyed to Ottawa to witness the signing of the agreement.

The question then became who would be the right person to direct the new facility. Benson Estambale was not an HIV specialist, but a microbiologist. His field was malaria and other, what he calls, "neglected diseases like bilharzia"— which is a parasitic disease (also known as schistosomiasis) picked up from snails in places like Lake Victoria. So, in 2004, when the University of Nairobi approached their professor of microbiology to take on this new job, he says that he was surprised. "I knew all the people who were part of the collaboration, but I was in a different field. My education was from Liverpool and Copenhagen; while the others were going to Canada and Washington, I had been travelling to Belgium and London," says Estambale. Yet, the job was his, a moment he describes as "the turning point of my life." In life, he told me, "there are moments of extreme excitement and moments of extreme fear. For me, that was both."

Estambale, who was fifty years old at the time, admits to not even being certain what his job was supposed to be. He went from official to official at the university asking, "what is it that I am to do?" His best advice came eventually from a colleague-superior who told him to go to the best furniture shop in Nairobi and identify what he wanted. Order top-of-the-line office furniture, he was told. "I was shocked, but he told me, once this international institute gets going the money will be coming in and 800,000 KSh ($10,000 CDN) will seem like nothing. The director will be seeing important visitors, and we don't need to be seen with shoddy things; he can't sign important agreements while sitting behind a school desk," says Estambale. What the whole thing really meant for Estambale, though, was the furthering of a long-held dream to realize at home the kind of centre of excellence he had experienced in the United Kingdom and Europe. This would be another step toward Africa controlling its destiny and future.

In 2002 the University of Manitoba's international liaison officer, Stella Hryniuk, flew to Nairobi to sit in on the annual meeting of the collaborators. Her report on the visit was glowing in general, with a section near the end devoted to the group's business meeting, where, chaired by King Holmes, project directors and project managers, principal investigators and representatives of the collaborating institutions (the universities of Manitoba, Illinois, Washington, Nairobi, and Ghent) could chew over what lay in store for the foreseeable future. While acknowledging progress in many areas, they shared, as well, a list of challenges. These included:

1. Breastfeeding transmission: the basic research was done and documented, but the question remained what to do with the knowledge?

2. Where might the work on vaccine development go?

3. Male circumcision trials were well-designed and the preliminary results impressive, but what to do next?

4. More microbicide trials were coming to confirm the efficacy of those antibiotics.

5. Diaphragm studies, a whole new area of research, were beginning.

6. HIV perinatal transmission studies by the collaborative group were defining the field, as few such studies are done in the West.

7. Operational research/system issues remained, especially the realization that more applied research was needed and the results of that research needed to be made part of Kenya's national public health programs and strategies for dealing with HIV/AIDS.

8. A variety of issues involving men: getting the attention of males in order to prevent the infection of wives and children by infected men; priorities of infected men for the use of antiretroviral drugs in such families; plans of infected men for their children when these become orphans; how the news media could be used to get to men on these issues.[1]

The attendees went on to worry as well about stubborn questions like why HIV/AIDS incidence continued to rise despite, at that time, two full decades of available preventive tools and resources; why antiretroviral treatments were (at the time) still so difficult and expensive to obtain; what public health training and research could best address future needs? Kenyans at the meeting still talked about the social stigma that HIV/AIDS occasioned in Kenyan society. The high cost of formula was cited as an obstacle in the strategy around less breast-feeding.

A decade later, the central matters of concern have not changed for the collaboration. They remain the stubborn questions that preoccupy everybody; the only difference is that the people addressing these matters now are a new generation of researchers. All the young scientists, doctors, and nurses who populated the conference halls at the January 2010 annual meeting in Nairobi (see Chapter 1), learning about and discussing progress on all fronts and looking at the future—theirs is now the partnership and theirs are the challenges.

Allan Ronald once itemized the ideals of the partnership between the Kenyans and the outsider Canadians, Americans, and Europeans as, firstly, originating from the principle of being good guests. These would be the kind who bring part of the meal, clean up after themselves, and are sincerely interested in the host's stories. "Always remember," he would say as a kind of mantra with such regularity it couldn't help but became instilled, "we are visitors." The second ideal of the partnership was to train Kenyans and push for them to occupy the top positions in their country's health system. The hosts who had welcomed the outsiders deserved, as their part of the bargain, the best training where and when they needed it, and that they would be advanced to positions of responsibility the very moment they were ready to take that responsibility on. If the project didn't do this, it did nothing; educating young Kenyans was the key to sustainability.

Third on Ronald's list was the aim that everybody involved would adhere to science in its purest sense. "The reason we're there and the reason we're working together is to do the best science possible," Ronald would say. Theirs was not some soft-headed do-gooder program, neither was it foreign aid; it was, rather, an opportunity to apply time-tempered methodologies of rationality to difficult medical problems and puzzles. The promise of science would be backed by up-to-date training and equipment, but the important thing was rigorous adherence to the scientific method: maintaining open minds, investigating and testing properly, and having reason and rationality behind the end results. "That in itself is relevant to development," Ronald would say, meaning that a trained cadre of expertise—with respect for expertise and the methodology of expertise—is the foundation of functioning, modern, productive societies. Finally, according to the maxims, the collaboration believed in collaboration. This would not be a trite truism, but a continual negotiation to ensure that what everybody did in both the short term and the long haul would be an exercise of partnership. The worst thing Ronald could imagine was that his group of foreign scientists would get the label "freezer bandits" or "safari scientists"—those who use their marketable skills as researchers or investigators to head into exotic corners of the globe for their own aggrandizement. Nobody needed to be reminded that this exploitive version of scientific research was easy to do, and in fact getting easier. Africa, and particularly high-profile diseases like HIV/AIDS, had become glamorous to a certain set of footloose adventurers, and the grant pools were increasingly open to almost any plausible proposal. Too many were tempted by their own needs for adventure without leaving behind any benefits for the host country. But not these foreigners; they left something behind.

The experience and reputation developed in the Nairobi collaboration caught the attention of the wider world. In 1997, Plummer was asked by Prabhat Jha, a fellow Canadian who was then a World Bank official, to make a presentation about the importance of targeted interventions to key government leaders in India involved in the design of the second phase of that country's National AIDS Control Program. India had been spared the kind of epidemic that had hit Africa, but Indian authorities were still worried. And after witnessing the crisis in Africa, they were savvy enough to understand that limited energy and resources needed to be strictly directed to the places where they would do the most good. At the request of the World Bank and the Indian government, Plummer, along with Stephen Moses, James Blanchard, Allan Ronald, and Mark Tyndall, visited India to share their experience and expertise on focussing HIV preventive interventions on high-risk populations.

The resulting project became known as the India-Canada Collaborative HIV/AIDS Project (ICHAP).[2] Funded by CIDA, it ran from 2001 to 2006, and was based in the Indian states of Karnataka and Rajasthan. ICHAP worked with state-level governments to build capacity for designing and implementing HIV/AIDS prevention and control programs and developed six demonstration projects in the two states, focussing on program models for HIV prevention, care, and support for vulnerable populations, particularly in rural areas. Their growing experience was put to further use in 2002, when scientists from the University Manitoba, a group led by James Blanchard, were asked to assist the government of Pakistan to develop a comprehensive program of secondary surveillance for HIV/AIDS and sexually transmitted infections in that country.

In the middle of 2003, a design team from the newly formed Bill and Melinda Gates Foundation's India AIDS Initiative (known as "Avahan") visited ICHAP, and asked the Manitobans and their Indian colleagues to prepare a proposal to scale up HIV preventive interventions in the state of Karnataka as part of the Avahan program. By December, the funds from the Gates Foundation came through, and in collaboration with the Karnataka State AIDS Prevention Society, the University of Manitoba team became the executing agency for a large-scale HIV prevention project among high-risk populations in Karnataka state. HIV prevention programs and services were provided to over 60,000 female sex workers and over 20,000 men who were having sex with men. Stephen Moses, with his wife Jan, relocated to India in 2006 to direct the HIV/AIDS program there. Based in Bangalore in south India, the program evolved to become active in several states, managing a large portfolio of projects funded by a variety of local and international agencies.

Allan Ronald, for his part, retired from the University of Manitoba in 2000, but promptly teamed up with a group of medical people led by the University of Utah's Merle Sande and the pharmaceutical giant Pfizer to create an organization they called the Academic Alliance for AIDS Care and Prevention in Africa. Academic Alliance then, at the invitation of the school of medicine at Makerere University in Uganda, helped establish an infectious disease institute. Ronald and his wife Myrna set up residence in Kampala for three years to get things started, training physicians, nurses, clinical officers, behavioural scientists, clinical investigators, and lab technicians. By 2010, the institute had seen almost 6,000 health care workers from twenty-seven African countries pass through its training program, all in the service of better addressing AIDS as well as other infectious diseases. The links of the Nairobi collaboration now reached worldwide, the participants travelling as far as airplanes would fly them and as far as their interests could imagine.

All this had not unfolded seamlessly. Indeed, there had been bumps along the way. The Nairobi collaboration had no roadmap to follow, it had to create the roadmap. Working backwards, it is possible to view the development of the project of the three foreign universities in Kenya, and in particular the University of Manitoba, as something that got invented as it went along. It wasn't fitted into a pre-existing mould; it was created out of the passions of the personnel who were involved in it, meeting the urgencies of the needs on the ground. All three universities, Washington, Ghent, and Manitoba supplied sorts of expeditionary forces that took themselves off to faraway Africa. Like such armies might have functioned throughout history, they were forced to improvise and live by their wits. For the history of the project to be different, it would have meant having entire systems of support at the levels of the granting agencies that undergirded international (or what has now become known as global) health research, as well as different systems in the universities themselves. Thirty years later, people talk about global health and some mechanisms are in place. They weren't in 1980. Now, the University of Manitoba has a staff director for external relations who reports to the president, has made trips to Kenya, and has met with Kenyan officials. In 1980 no such official existed. These structures and processes were invented because of the activities of the expeditionary force who had, in many senses, to pave the way. But while they were doing so, they went without the kinds of supports that in retrospect would have been tremendously helpful.

Kelly MacDonald itemizes the complaints. "We didn't have the supports from home to actually get the work done," she says. "In Canada we didn't have a mechanism through CIHR to award our institutions the kind of programmatic support that we needed." At the institutional level, the University of Manitoba is a medium-sized institution without the kind of endowment that some universities are blessed with. It did not, therefore, have the deep pockets to say, "okay we're going to cover you while you do this work". On top of that, it didn't really occur to anyone there that this should be its job. This, according to MacDonald, compromised the researchers' ability to compete in the big-league world in which they were playing. " It was really hard to have to watch people from other institutions where they had money to burn when we couldn't afford even things like petrol for the vehicles to get down to the clinic," says MacDonald. "Other people would be flying all over the world with their liquid nitrogen tanks. It was really frustrating trying to decide whether we would spend our last 500 bucks on fetal bovine serum, or to buy liquid nitrogen to ship the stuff home."

Arnold Naimark, who was president of the University of Manitoba during the opening years of the Nairobi project, says that the university was "enormously proud" of the growing achievements of the work and calls them a "jewel in the crown" of the university. The administration, it is true, supported the project by allowing people whose salaries the university was paying to go off to Kenya for extended periods of time. But when there were difficulties, he admits to watching from a distance as those more closely involved tried to work things out. Yet when Allan Ronald in 2008 got a hint that the top tier of Manitoba researchers, by then well-known across the world of science, were being head-hunted by bigger and wealthier institutions, he fired off a letter to his own university president,

Emőke Szathmáry, who responded promptly assuring everybody that no one would be poached during her watch.

Occasionally, things were handled downright badly. Something that emerged to hover like a cloud over the story of the project was the bumpiness of its relationship with one of its significant funders, CIDA. In the early years, the project worked hard to woo this major governmental source of foreign aid, only to be told repeatedly that CIDA's mandate did not let it finance medical research. Eventually, the collaboration tailored a project for education and AIDS awareness with heavy involvement by Kenyans, led by Elizabeth Ngugi. The Strengthening STD/HIV Control In Kenya made it through the vetting process and received substantial support, $1 million a year for five years with the possibility to renew when that term was up (see Chapter 3). But the relationship, though the program went on for almost fifteen years, was prone to hiccups that left the participants frequently rattled. The final episode saw the Canadian agency abruptly cutting support in 2004 with about a year still left on the clock. The program had weathered a first round of CIDA budget cutting in 1996 but was not so lucky a decade later.

There remains a fair amount of mystification and second-guessing around what exactly went wrong with a project CIDA had referred to in earlier publicity as a "landmark project" for the agency. One explanation was that there were personality clashes between officials back in Ottawa and the staff in Nairobi. But that can't be the whole story. Likewise, the explanation that things soured because of a culture clash between a bureaucratic agency with one set of agendas and a university-backed project with another doesn't tell the entire story either, though it comes closer and does offer some insight. In short, a lot of people felt hurt and betrayed and still nurse bitterness years later. "CIDA treated us like bandits," says Plummer. "I don't think they ever realized what they had." What he means is that the broad value of the Nairobi program should have outweighed anything else. It is worth, therefore, trying to understand what might have gone wrong, not least because doing so can provide a cautionary tale about what can go awry, and at how many levels, between those out in the field and those who wield the purse strings thousands of kilometers away.

When it was cancelled, the CIDA grant was into its third phase, having been running for almost fifteen years. During this phase, arguably its last, those managing the program (at this point Chester Morris and Ngugi) were supposed to demonstrate how the services they had developed were going to be off-loaded onto other, on the ground NGOs. CIDA was always adamant that they wanted to provide start-up funding, not keep projects going in perpetuity. The problem,

Joanne Embree believes, is that off-loading didn't look promising and CIDA realized this. The letter detailing the end of CIDA's grant for the program was sent from project manager Evelyn Voigt to the University of Manitoba's executive director for international relations, Jim Gardner, on July 30, 2004. It cites an opinion from a monitor's report that "conditions for Project sustainability do not exist," and chides the project for failing to move "from being an implementer to being a catalyst." Though the University of Nairobi eventually did establish a Centre for HIV Prevention as per its aims, and solid funding from a number of sources ultimately materialized to keep the project going, the letter is firm in its skepticism that this would ever happen. Most substantially, though, it takes the University of Manitoba and project management to task for some business issues: "irregularities in asset procurement, importation and ownership," "misuse of the MOU between the Government of Canada and Kenya in purchasing assets," and "potential irregularities in staff time charged to the Project".

It took a while to reach this final impasse. Embree was, by this time, head of microbiology at the University of Manitoba. The first rumbles of difficulty came as early as 2002 when senior people in the university management took her aside to tell her something was afoot. But it was difficult to be specific about exactly what. Was it that the personality or culture clashes were perhaps now rising to the surface? In brief, the Strengthening STD/HIV Control program was initiated by a generation of CIDA staff both in Nairobi and Ottawa who were excited by the ideas it encompassed and were, therefore, determined to find ways to make it work even if, as Embree puts it, this required "pounding round pegs into square holes." A decade later, those staff both in Ottawa and in Nairobi had retired or moved on. The new crop exemplified the other side of the coin: not taking something you think is important and figuring out how to make it work, but taking something you've decided not to like and figuring out how to put an end to it. Once they were in this mood, says Embree, CIDA became "suspicious of all kinds of things we were doing, including that the money might be being spent on 'research'—as if that was a dirty word." There is no denying that things descended to nasty levels, with lawyers and legal threats. The university, Embree says gratefully, threw its support "100 percent behind the project" with staff from high up in the president's office having regular meetings with CIDA officials.

Larry Gelmon tries to provide some perspective from the project side on what got CIDA alarmed, shedding light on the culture clash and matters that left the project vulnerable. Things, he admits, started informally and loosely, which spilled over into bookkeeping. It was, again, the "money into the common pot" tendency. "If money was coming in," says Gelmon, "it would be put into a general pot, and from that pot salaries were paid, vehicles were purchased, travel was done. And there wasn't a lot of distinction between various projects." This is what is known in the business as "basket funding," and can arguably be a good way for a research project to operate, providing perhaps the most efficient spending of public tax dollars, mainly because items are only purchased when they are absolutely necessary. "The money was shepherded like it was gold and certainly nobody used any for personal gain," declares Embree. However, such a system clashed head-on with changes that were happening back in Ottawa.

By the late 1990's, the Canadian government's accounting culture had changed dramatically, with accountability and strict line-item fiscal responsibility gaining ascendancy over almost all other considerations in all departments. That this trumped all else was underlined for scientists out in the field when the agency got rid of technical advisors. Where previously CIDA had listened to medical specialists on its staff, now it was only development specialists. "This," says Gelmon, "caused a gap where they (CIDA) didn't have the capability to understand what we were trying to do. Now it was only financial people. The auditors would come and say 'you bought a vehicle from the budget of this project but gave it to that; this person's salary came from five different projects'. The perception arose in CIDA that we were financially irresponsible…and we were wasting the Canadian taxpayer's money."

Sorting matters out was complicated and took a couple of years. Eventually, ownership of project vehicles was transferred to the organizations that had purchased them, and all duties owing were paid. "But we got hammered," reiterates Gelmon. "We spent two years chasing down owners to get vehicles re-registered, vehicles that CIDA argued were still Canadian government property. In the end, although everything was put right, a sour taste remained that never really disappeared."

As a footnote, it seems more than slightly ironic that the program money that sustained the Nairobi collaboration through the first decade of the twenty-first century was largely not Canadian by source. In September 2010, the group received over $20 million dollars from PEPFAR to extend HIV prevention work among most at-risk populations, expanding to new sites in Nairobi, as well as two other Kenyan provinces. As with the work on male circumcision it turned out to be agencies in other countries, primarily the United States, that recognized the value of the Canadian enterprise and provided substantial financial support to expand the scope of activities.

That was all now in the past. Thirty years on, it was time for a generational change. That the project had gone as it had—for the most part overwhelmingly well—had a lot to do with personnel. And with the luck of the personnel that got either attracted or recruited. There is a certain genius behind finding the right people, and the Nairobi project had some good luck in that department. Many say that it started with Allan Ronald. Ronald had a theory of teaching that involved keeping your eyes open—not unlike a hockey or baseball scout—for the prospective scientist as yet unformed in the youngster who comes through your door. And then not letting them get away. "In every medical school class," he reflects, "there are ten to fifteen students who could become good scientists. The job is to figure out who those are. You listen to the questions they ask, you try to understand what turns them on. If you get the right people, they return ten dollars for every dollar you put in."

But by 2010 a number of the senior members of the collaboration were moving, one by one, to more settled positions back in North America and Europe—though two of them, Frank Plummer and King Holmes, kept actively interested, continuing to supervise some of their charges and projects in Nairobi. Plummer still held a Gates Foundation Grand Challenge grant to continue work on HIV vaccine research for the next eight years. But his main work was back in Canada where he headed up the National Microbiology Laboratory, in charge of examining dangerous pathogens and controlling potential epidemics for Canada's Public Health Agency. King Holmes, after seventeen years as director of the University of Washington's Center for AIDS and Sexually Transmitted Diseases, was given a new job in 2006 (and at age sixty-eight), chair of the university's department of global health. A third mainstay of the early collaboration, Peter Piot, who had spent more than a decade as executive director of UNAIDS in Geneva, by 2010 was about to take a new position as director of the London School of Hygiene and Tropical Medicine. This historic institution, a branch of the University of London based in Bloomsbury, boasted almost 4,000 students from more than a hundred countries and is recognized as the leading public health and global health facility in Britain, if not the world. On the Kenyan side, Herbert Nsanze was now semi-retired in Uganda, his home country. Hannington Pamba had died, as had Job Bwayo, murdered in a violent car-jacking. Others from the original group, like J.O. Ndinya-Achola, who had been a steady partner in both Nairobi and Kisumu, still showed up at his office, but was less and less in the front lines of things. He also suffered health problems, and in early 2011 passed away.

So, in Nairobi, the next generation were the ones to watch. The trainees had become the scientists, and some of these—those everybody still referred to as "young scientists"—were in fact already at mid-career, with many months or years of travel back and forth between their home bases and Kenya under their belts. The University of Washington's Grace John-Stewart first went to Nairobi in 1993 and lived there until 2005. Her interests then were maternal health studies around HIV-positive women and breast-feeding, and that is what continues to absorb her. After 2005, John-Stewart continued making two to three trips per year between Seattle and Nairobi to collaborate with colleagues there.[3] Their project was dedicated to work on prevention of mother-to-child transmission of HIV, molecular epidemiology studies, studies of co-infections such as tuberculosis and HIV, and pediatric studies. Other University of Washington scientists included Scott Mc-Clelland, who led the Mombasa research site, and Jared Baeton, an epidemiologist and specialist in the organization of clinical trials on HIV interventions.

Among the Canadians, those keeping up the work on Plummer's eight-year-long, $15 million research project on the quest for an HIV vaccine included Keith Fowke, Blake Ball, and Rupert Kaul, all of them former trainees and fellows, now increasingly prominent as scientists in their own right. New names, too numerous to list, appeared almost monthly at one level or another of the research chain: Kenyans, Swedes, Americans, Canadians; the prominent young Canadians including gynecologist Lisa Avery, microbiologist Lyle MacKinnon, and Marissa Becker, a public health specialist whose field was care for vulnerable populations.

For all of them, the nerve centre of their Nairobi world would be the new building where, one morning, Maureen Njoga pointed a visitor to the wall-mounted chart that outlined the current state of the collaboration. Five clinics in three different shantytowns plus a drop-in centre for midtown sex workers supported HIV/AIDS prevention work as well as testing, counselling, and distribution of antiretroviral therapies. Maureen and the visitor needed to dodge because traffic along the corridor was bustling. Down the hall they located offices for project director Larry Gelmon and the clinical director Joshua Kimani, both of them under pressure to keep the pieces in place to sustain an enterprise that now has eighty-five staff. This, it might be pointed out, is global health in action. Global health is now not just a term, it has offices and laboratories and money. It has its department in Seattle at the University of Washington; it has a presence in increasing numbers of medical faculties across the world. In Winnipeg, a brass plate bolted to the door of a suite of rooms in the medical school announced, in 2009, the establishment of its Centre for Global Health. And it was high time. In the course of a decade, more than a $100 million from various foundations had flowed through the University of Manitoba to support the projects in India, China, Pakistan, as well as Kenya. This very substantial sum supported everything from service delivery programs in HIV/AIDS prevention to maternal child health, as well as training and research. An optimist—which is what everybody involved both now and over thirty years has had to be—might believe that the Canadian health minister's words, that the best response to perils that don't respect borders is ensuring that our knowledge and action also transcend geographic boundaries, seemed actually possible.

AIDS World

The short history of the African AIDS epidemic—certainly from the perspective of researchers based in Nairobi—looks something like this:

In 1984, researchers worked in facilities so basic that there was not even a proper serological test available to help them identify HIV, the new virus confronting them. Determining someone's infection involved sending a sample of blood to Europe or America and waiting for weeks or months. By observation, however, the researchers in Nairobi believed that what they were seeing in Kenya was the same disease being reported in North America, in San Francisco, New York, and Vancouver. In North America, the prevailing mindset was that the new virus was confined to gay men and that heterosexual transmission was a rare exception. Yet, once the results of the study conducted with Nairobi sex workers came back at the end of 1985, everybody realized that the virus could be transmitted equally well heterosexually and that there was potential for an epidemic in East Africa, certainly among sex workers.

By 1990, researchers in Africa had a good sense of how big the problem was, and had some very firm ideas about how it might be controlled and its spread prevented. The minimum elements of this strategy included aggressively treating all STDs; persuading men to use condoms at least when they were with sex workers; persuading HIV-infected mothers not to breast-feed their babies, or at least to limit breast-feeding; and encouraging men to get circumcised. The first paper that linked male circumcision and HIV had been published in 1988. Such specific strategies, those who advocated them believed, would reduce HIV transmission several fold. AIDS, by this time, was universally recognized as a huge problem everywhere in Africa, but it was frustrating to note how hard it still was to get the message out. The question remained: "here's the problem and here's what causes it… What are we going to do about it?"

By 1998, AIDS was devastating the continent of Africa, yet the epidemic was still not getting the kind of attention most felt it urgently needed. A great deal of bureaucracy had been developed around the epidemic, but proper prevention and care services were insufficiently delivered. Science had made some inroads on treatment: in North America, the first drug cocktails shown to prolong the lives of those infected had been miraculously developed and were available. But a year's worth of the medications cost $12,000, so were seen as little use to impoverished Africa. Politically, there were pushes by activists like Stephen Lewis and concerned voices like U.S. President Bill Clinton for more investment in these antiretroviral drugs and in getting them out to people in poor countries. The downside was that the campaign to treat those infected with HIV/AIDS overshadowed efforts at preventing the disease. Optimism about development of a vaccine remained high, but even that momentum was overshadowed by the treatment campaigns. After the trial for the vaccine developed by Oxford in 1999 was abandoned as a failure in 2005, discouragement set in.

In 2005, after a court case in South Africa that permitted the distribution of generic drugs from India, the price of antiretrovirals came down. As a result, some became available in Africa and agitation to distribute them grew more fervent. On the other side, prevention was still not sufficiently funded or promoted.

In 2012, we now have a much greater understanding of how treatment can lead to prevention. Antiretroviral treatments not only prolong lives, but also inhibit (though not entirely) the infectiousness of a person carrying HIV. Yet prevention still is not keeping pace with new infections, and the strategies that were identified in 1990 are still not being implemented at a sufficient scale. Strategies and goals around prevention are still urgently required. The cornerstones of this approach for Africa, many recognize, will be a future where condoms are used in all high-risk sexual encounters, where access to testing is available for all, and where most males get circumcised.

First, the bad news: at the start of the second decade of the twenty-first century, thirty years after the first identified cases of HIV/AIDS, the epidemic in sub-Saharan Africa, by far too many objective indices, remains a losing battle. True, more and more people are on life-prolonging antiretroviral therapies, something that mushroomed when costs dropped from $12,000 per year per patient to $100 with the arrival of generic drugs and when donors to purchase them sprang into action. Yet for every 100 people who are put on antiretroviral therapies each year, southern Africa registers 250 new HIV infections. The battle of prevention—to stop new infections—is not even close to being turned. Globally, 2 million people continue to die each year from AIDS, but 3 million are newly infected. In a 2010 interview with the *New York Times*, such disheartening statistics forced Peter Piot to concede that "in 2003 we were at a tipping point in the right direction, now I'm afraid we're at a tipping point in the wrong direction."[1] What he worried about was a combination of increasing infection rates with fatigue on the part of those financing and organizing what few control measures were succeeding. How much longer would the donor money continue to flow? It was like the little boy in the Netherlands with his finger in the dike, but the finger was getting tired and the dike was under assault from more and more water.

It would be irredeemably harsh to the dedicated labours of tens of thousands who have been working tirelessly on every aspect of the epidemic to declare that the fight against AIDS in Africa has been a failure. Yet, it is likewise impossible to declare it a success. The battle is far from won and—worse—shows only sporadic and fleeting signs that it is even winnable. In 2004, the editor of the *Lancet* lamented twenty years of failure in the quest for an AIDS vaccine, a project Richard Horton described as "chasing a chimera. The virus can run faster than the human immune system and much faster than our technical capabilities in vaccine research."[2] AIDS always has been dreadful disease. Once it gets hold of a victim and the disease develops, one suffers a miserable death as the immune system shuts down, ceasing to guard from other illnesses and infections. The question remained, though, did it need to be an epidemic, as it was for a decade among gay men in North America and continues to be in sub-Saharan Africa? Did it have to kill millions of people and cripple entire countries on continents like Africa, or could it have been nipped in the bud? What was or wasn't done; what mistakes were made; what strategies and attitudes would have been necessary in order to stop AIDS in its tracks? It took a long time for the world to confront such painful questions. Yet to pose them is a brave act, for engaging in the ensuing discussion means having to confront not just hypothetical but real failures, which have cost millions of lives.

At the 2008 International AIDS Conference in Mexico City, the seventeenth such global conference attended religiously by those working on HIV/AIDS, the atmosphere was infected by this sombre sense of failure. Stefano Bertozzi, the man who had worked on HIV prevention for the host country, Mexico, for several years, bluntly lamented that "billions of dollars have been spent on what should have been an easily preventable disease." The editor of the *Lancet* acknowledged the frittering away of time and energies by noting that the world had been "diverted from a long-term prevention response by believing that a single technological fix might solve all the problems." The fix he meant was either the vaccine that still hasn't come or a cure, which antiretroviral therapy, for all its benefits to AIDS sufferers, is not. The brutal facts seemed to haunt everybody; after 30 million deaths, 2.7 million new infections still occur each year. Once the discussion opened up, people turned it in on themselves. The ABCs of abstinence, being faithful, and using condoms seemed almost an embarrassment, condemned now by one congress participant for "infantilizing prevention."

The blunt conclusion come to by Frank Plummer, when he looks back on the almost three decades of AIDS in Africa, is that prevention strategies that should have been obvious were not vigorously pursued. It is a severe assessment, bound to leave much discomfort among those in charge of public policy. Plummer acknowledges, first, that those who would have prevented the disease from turning into a raging epidemic actually held a lot of cards in their hands, important among them the knowledge that, despite prevailing perceptions, it is actually quite difficult to acquire HIV infection. "It is inefficiently transmitted," he says, emphasizing the fact that probabilities of transmission lie in the range of much less than 1 percent, even with an infected heterosexual partner, provided that male partners are circumcised and that you don't have pre-exiting STDs. This means that, although HIV seems to have spread rapidly, had high-risk groups been aggressively and effectively targeted, preventative strategies would have had some time in which to do their work. "AIDS," Plummer says, "should have been easily stopped before the epidemic became what it did. That we were not able to do it was a colossal failure of public health."

Another succinct critic of how the epidemic was handled is Elizabeth Pisani. Pisani has a PhD in infectious disease epidemiology from the London School of Hygiene and Tropical Medicine and, for a decade, worked providing research, analysis, and policy advice to UNAIDS, the WHO, the World Bank, and the CDC, as well as to the ministries of health of China, Indonesia, East Timor, and the Philippines. Then she wrote a book, *The Wisdom of Whores*. Her thesis is that politics and political correctness have consistently stood in the way of HIV prevention. Prevention would have been achieved by aggressively and effectively targeting two groups of people across the world: commercial sex workers and intravenous drug users who potentially share needles. Pisani is particularly harsh when assessing Africa. "Africa," she writes, "is a giant, in-your-face failure for the HIV prevention industry. It might be even worse without our prevention efforts, though it is hard to see how it could be. On the prevention balance sheet, we're in the red to the tune of 45 million infections. In some countries, over 80 percent of all adults will die of HIV."[3]

The purpose of epidemiology is to contain and, at the very best, combined with public health services, prevent epidemics. Much was made, however, of the fact that HIV/AIDS, right from its inception, differed from any other epidemic. Those proposing this danced between explanations and excuses. HIV, for one thing, is a virus that mutates rapidly, making it exceedingly challenging to bring it to ground with a vaccine. The epidemic also occurred within a complicated social and cultural context, striking first in the gay communities of New York and San Francisco, where men passed it to other men, then attacking the needle-using drug culture worldwide, and then heterosexuals in Africa. Sex and drugs are two things that in almost every culture are sensitive topics, and messing with them is a delicate business. So people and their governments became careful to the point of reticence. Dealing head-on with HIV/AIDS was touchy on at least two fronts. First, there is enough lingering puritanism to ensure that sexual and drug-taking lifestyles are unapproachable without stigmatizing. In the last decades of the twentieth century, nobody wanted to appear judgmental, least of all official agencies. Yet at the same time, society is sufficiently judgmental to make practitioners of gay sex, or drug using, or even heterosexually promiscuous lifestyles, wary. Fear of stigmatization caused people to want to hide their infection or even not want to know their HIV status. The authorities bent over backwards to let people know their lifestyles were not the business of the authorities, but became less like true epidemiologists who have to name things for what they are, and more like social workers not wishing to cause offence. They chose to protect vulnerable people from moral judgment, notwithstanding that moral judgment was not the issue, public health safety was.

The point that Pisani makes firmly is the one that dogged the reaction to HIV/AIDS from the very beginning: standard practices of epidemiology on the one side, and human rights on the other, became pitched as contradictory positions. "Public health is inherently a somewhat fascist discipline," she writes. "It protects the health of the many." She uses SARS, the virus that landed squarely in Canada in 2003, as an example. When SARS emerged, there was no hesitation to restrict people's movements, force people to be tested, and register them if they were infected. Whole cities (including Canada's biggest city, Toronto) were virtually shut down. The practices initiated for SARS adhered to a pattern going back to the nineteenth century, when many countries registered people with syphilis and did not hesitate to ask those people about their sex partners. Once identified, the partners were tracked down and offered testing and treatment. In the course of that effort, Pisani points out, no one complained much, even though syphilis was at one time every bit as stigmatized as HIV/AIDS is now. But HIV/AIDS somehow got cast as different. When authorities in the United States, Sweden, or the German state of Bavaria tried to use the same measures that had been used on syphilis against HIV/AIDS early in the epidemic, people complained and many key measures were quashed. "AIDS focused people's attention on the rights of people living with an infectious disease. This was a new departure in public health, and a welcome change in many ways," Pisani writes. "But the fear of violating people's perceived rights overrode many otherwise routine principles of public health. By the time we began trying to address HIV in Africa, mandatory HIV testing and contact tracing were philosophically out of the question. Completely confidential and strictly voluntary HIV testing were the order of the day."[4]

A sort of skewed conventional wisdom developed that came to accept that, since HIV testing would expose people to stigmatization, routine testing was considered dubious and compulsory testing was labelled an outright evil. Astoundingly, HIV/AIDS was for a long time singled out as one of the only sexually transmitted diseases that did not, in the United States, require reporting to health authorities. By 2010, this had changed: HIV/AIDS cases were being reported to local health boards by physicians and sexual partners were to be informed that they were at risk for developing and spreading the disease. But that was nearly thirty years on in the epidemic.[5] A second notable issue about the HIV/AIDS epidemic was that very early on the victims of the disease and those championing their interests got hold of the agenda and ran with it. This was not a bad thing, in that the victims of such a serious disease, be they gay Americans, people addicted to intravenous drugs, or middle-aged heterosexual Africans, should never be ignored or marginalized. But what happened was that the needs of victims, whether that was treatment or protection from embarrassment and stigmatization, became the drivers, elbowing out measures and strategies that might have contained the epidemic. Frank Plummer observes that the lobby that always commanded the floor at the global HIV/AIDS meetings was of people who were already infected. "There was never going to be," he says, "an equivalent lobby of people who didn't have HIV/AIDS—though they might get it." The lobby of those already infected demanded recognition, treatments, and such things as assured anonymity when they were tested. While this was good, some of these measures simultaneously worked against prevention strategies, either by diverting resources from condoms and education and circumcision or, more directly, by challenging what Pisani might have labelled "fascist" actions like mandatory testing and compulsory disclosures of sexual histories.

Those who spent a lot of time in Nairobi during those years have had to do their own soul-searching about how things might have been handled differently. King Holmes tells how the first impetus he encountered was to bring balance to what everybody knew was a complicated situation. "In the early days," says Holmes, "I was part of a group in our state of Washington that drafted regulations that said before you do any testing you had to have counselling, and that every-thing was voluntary." It became apparent before long, he admits, that these regula-tions were actually an impediment: the regulations designed to be sensitive and protect people's privacy discouraged both health care practitioners and at-risk patients from aggressively doing what they should have done. "Physicians either didn't have the time to go through all those steps our regulations demanded, or they were afraid that if they didn't do it right, they would get into legal trouble," he says. The unfortunate result, Holmes adds, is that testing of broad numbers of people didn't happen. Globally, there was the hope for a vaccine, but on the ground and locally there were few services for sex workers and a real effort to avoid saying much about preventing HIV. "We backed away from fear of stigma-tizing. Even today we are still not investing enough in prevention. We are clearly not treating our way out of it and we are falling farther and farther behind."

It didn't have to be this way. Frank Plummer makes an adamant case that the strategies to dramatically slow, if not entirely prevent, the spread of HIV/AIDS had all been identified by the late 1980s. Those in the front lines of research knew then that HIV is transmitted most easily when it comes into contact with sores, lesions, or a foreskin. So one solution became obvious: Screen for sexually transmitted infections and treat them among women, men, and transgendered people who sell sex, and among their clients and regular partners. For hetero-sexuals in most of the world (Africa included) the highest-risk sex is that which is paid for, so the solution is to create incentives to use condoms every time sex is bought or sold. In communities where there is lots of HIV, circumcise men. None of these strategies were engaged nearly as effectively as they should have been, with the result that the epidemic still rages. "What should have been done in 1990 to attack and prevent the spread of AIDS," Plummer says, "still needs to be done now." For his part, King Holmes believes that for prevention, what is needed is a multi-component strategy that would deal with a variety of factors such as discordant couples (those where one partner is infected with HIV while the other is not—and may not even know the status of their partner), early-access antiretroviral therapy, circumcision, and condoms.

For a long time, difficulties in the battle against the HIV/AIDS epidemic were framed as a question of money. Those who were critical blamed the West for stinginess. This still happens. In the lead up to the G8/G20 summit in Toronto in June 2010, a lead article in the *Globe and Mail* newspaper pointed out the shortcomings of the G8 leaders' promises to pay for HIV/AIDS treatments in Africa five years earlier when, at their meeting in Gleneagles, Scotland, the same group promised unwavering support for the continent. "The Promise," as the headline screamed, was that every HIV/AIDS patient would have access to life-saving medicine by 2010. That not all of them got it was posed as just another broken promise that threatens the lives of millions of Africans with HIV. The newspaper asked, will it be any different this time around?[6]

The reality, numbers-wise, was as the journalist writing the article made it out to be. Thirty-three million people were infected with HIV, the great majority of them in southern Africa. Far from all of those who required it received the antiretroviral therapies that would keep them alive. The numbers of those contracting the virus annually continued to exceed the number of those going on antiretroviral therapies. But whether it was all a problem of money was a much too complicated question to dismiss easily. HIV/AIDS is a disease that in fact receives the lion's share of health monies in many developing countries. In Kenya, it uses up 60 percent of the government health budget. In 2001, according to Peter Piot, global expenditure on AIDS rose dramatically, reaching $15 billion a year by 2010. "This is serious money," he noted. The problem was not lack of money per se, but far more insidious concerns like potential donor fatigue and inefficiency of the distribution of both money and services. On the one hand, as success against AIDS remained elusive, arguments to transfer resources back into fights against other highly visible and equally deadly diseases like malaria and tuberculosis gained strength. On the other hand was the sense that all that money was not reaching its proper targets. "Against AIDS we should be doing better with the same amount of money," Piot speculated.[7] Efficiency in the use of such vast amounts of money was, in fact, a great challenge.

In 2001, the UN General Assembly in New York convened a special session on HIV/AIDS, calling together thousands of experts—scientists, medical people, and government and civil society leaders—to identify what they believed it would take to fight the epidemic. A few months later the *Lancet* published what a group of HIV/AIDS experts believed the project might cost. Their estimate: $27 billion for a package of public health interventions, including condom promotion programs; mass media campaigns on television, radio, and billboards; HIV/AIDS education programs for schools, factories, and other businesses; HIV testing; and STD treatment services. Implementing all this would expand what was already happening in many places throughout the developing world through to 2010, though it did not include the many billions of additional dollars required for the medical care of HIV/AIDS patients.[8] Ten years earlier, steps to curtail the epidemic would have cost a great deal less. In 1990, the Nairobi researchers led by Stephen Moses undertook a cost-effectiveness study where they constructed a mathematical model predicated on 80 percent condom use by commercial sex workers and their clients. They concluded that such a strategy, if broadly implemented and adhered to, would cost about ten dollars per HIV infection prevented. This estimated the cost of each HIV infection prevented, assuming that each person who would have become infected would have infected, on average, one other person. It did not factor in effects that would come beyond that. Measured against the costs of treatment, ten dollars for each prevented infection was a bargain—and still is. Even though the costs of basic antiretroviral therapy have dropped to $100 a year per patient, that $100 does not include the costs of clinic services and delivery of the medication on a daily basis to patients, which increase the cost substantially. As is always the case, the cost of prevention is cheaper than the cost of cure—or in the case of HIV/AIDS, the cost of maintenance treatment.[9]

It was possible to stymie HIV/AIDS, and in some places they did just that. Uganda is a country of 32 million people, neighbour to the north and the west of Kenya. At the very beginning, Uganda had one of the worst HIV infection rates in all the world, an alarming 22 percent of its population. It was one of the first countries where HIV/AIDS showed up, and the country where University of Washington researcher Martina Morris's theories on concurrency, the sexual practice that invited transmission (see Chapter 2), were based. But very early, likewise, Uganda took steps to meet the crisis head-on.

In 1986, at the end of what had been a long and bloody civil war, the victorious Yoweri Museveni sent sixty officers from his "revolutionary movement forces" to Cuba for advanced training so that they might learn better how to hold on to the military success they had achieved. In due course, Fidel Castro sent Museveni a message warning him to beware of a danger as great or greater than counter-revolution. His sixty officers, upon arrival in Havana, had undergone routine HIV testing, and sixteen of them had turned up positive. Museveni, needless to say, was shocked. But unlike some of his fellow leaders in other countries, he did not retreat into defensiveness or denial. He took responsibility for the new disease, began making it the topic in all his speeches, and, according to observers, was able to speak with knowledge and authority.

Uganda rolled out a campaign to fight HIV/AIDS, with its directives coming right from the office of President Museveni. Gary Slutkin worked for the WHO Global Program on AIDS between 1987 and 1994, assisting the thirteen eastern and central southern African countries at the heart of the epidemic, and was the principal epidemiologist assigned to assist Uganda. "An intense program of public education, information, and skills building reached into every corner of the country," he recounts. "The program followed two sequential WHO-assisted plans and consisted of information and training channelled through twenty-six sectors of the country, from the military to women's groups to refugees to journalists and teachers."[10] It was as thorough an approach as any country could experience. Community-based workshops with information and education on changing risky behaviours were brought to almost every district. Within a few years, it paid off; Uganda saw its infection rates drop by 80 percent. Allan Ronald, who stayed in close touch with the Ugandan story during those years, describes how there was no skirting about causes of death in public obituaries as was the case in many other countries. "When you died, they said that you died of AIDS," says Ronald. The public saw AIDS right away, not as something to avoid talking about, but as a disease that, alarmingly, killed otherwise healthy people. Uganda welcomed the input of foreign NGOs, and saw to it that the message was not restricted to the capital, Kampala, but was taken into the countryside by agencies that set up peer-support systems in every small village. The message was put out to young people by the popular musician Philly Lutaaya, himself HIV-positive, who travelled from school to school. Ugandans started getting tested, then they almost spontaneously started changing their sexual habits from concurrency to something they colourfully called "zero grazing," as well as increasing condom use and delaying onset of first intercourse.

What happened in Uganda, one might think, should have become a model for all of Africa, if not the world. But to the frustration of many watching, this didn't happen. Other countries whose problems were just as serious—or at least about to become so—did not pick up Uganda's vigorous, all-encompassing approach. Slutkin complained that in spite of Uganda's success, its information, education, and communication program was never replicated anywhere else. But he was at a loss to explain why. "People," he could only conclude glumly, "resist doing what others have done."

One of the hallmarks of Uganda's success was, in the largest sense, how widely individuals embraced the responsibility for their own health. This is no small challenge in the battle against infectious diseases. People have to know the facts, and they have to know the severity of the threat they are facing. But then they too, not just the bureaucratic agencies, have to take responsibility. Yet, as those in the West have known for fifty years with cigarette smoking and its connection to lung cancer, achieving this is not an easy matter.

Astoundingly, disinformation remains rife a full generation after the arrival of AIDS. In 2010 in Nairobi, I met John. Thirty-two years old, John is something quite unusual in Kenya, a gay man who openly admits both to that and to being a sex worker. Homosexuality has long been anathema, something former president Daniel Arap Moi declared was "foreign, not done by Kenyans." Putting the lie to that, John, every day, rises early in the flat he shares with his boyfriend, showers, dresses, dabs on some Hugo Boss cologne, and then is ready. At an Internet café he will check out a gay website for tourists arriving and wanting to "hook up," then he cruises the streets looking for some business. Recent assignations, he told me, included a United Nations official whose wife was out of the country and a Christian pastor. But when we met, John admitted something both astonishing and depressing: despite his high-risk occupation and despite the fact that HIV/AIDS had been around almost his entire life, John did not know until a year earlier that he could get HIV through gay sex. John was not wilfully ignorant, but for a long and dangerous time, he was ignorant nevertheless and in a perilous position to be so. Now he knows that he carries the virus and for a long time, no doubt, spread it. Politically incorrect though such an observation may appear, it is numbing to see an epidemic enter its second generation saddled with as much superstition and downright ignorance—excusable or wilful—among those who are its victims. The responsibility of education rests squarely on governments, health and school officials, churches, and the media. But the responsibility to listen, learn, and behave rests on every individual and every family.

My encounter with John was at the Sex Worker Outreach Project (see Chapter 6). SWOP, covering the upper floor of a building on a commercial street in the middle of Nairobi, is one of the clinics under the umbrella of the Nairobi collaboration and is managed by social worker Gloria Gakii. There, where the walls are festooned with condoms and posters proclaiming tolerance and, most of all, safe sexual practices, John now carries out his other life, as a "peer leader" of fellow sex workers, doing his part to educate those who remain in the same position he used to be in. Most of the eighty to ninety people who pass through the doors each day are women, but a handful, like John, are young men. We watched a cross-section of clients lounging in the waiting room at mid-morning; about thirty women, some with small children. A few were young and strikingly attractive—college students trying to make extra cash. Others look a bit more hardened. Among them was Marion, a sturdy woman of thirty-five with a chipped front tooth who is, like John, a peer leader. To support herself and her ten-year-old son, Marion sells sex out of a "hot spot," a bar next to a mid-level hotel. In Marion's case, she had once studied at a college, worked in an office, and was married. But her husband beat her and she left; unable to find a job to support herself and her son, she turned to sex work. Dozens more clients pushed in, some to pick up their monthly dose of antiretroviral pills, some to obtain condoms, some to get HIV tests, the rapid test that now tells you your status in fifteen minutes. HIV testing is the first order of business at SWOP. But the lamentable thing, as John attests, is that even though they have been working the streets and bars for years, before SWOP, 80 percent of the clients had never had an HIV test. Once they get the test, they must live with the results, which is that 35 percent of them turn out to be HIV-positive. "The main job is to look after themselves as well as protect their clients," declared Gloria Gakii. If you discover you are negative, you want to keep it that way. Marion now insists on condoms, forgoing the fees that range from 500 to 3000 KSh (seven to forty-five dollars) if her clients refuse. Alternatively, if you are positive, as John turned out to be, you must protect your clients by using condoms, and save your own life by getting access to antiretroviral therapies.

For Marion and John, their attitudes and sense of responsibility have been altered. But it took a generation to reach this point—if we have in fact truly reached it. A disturbing story out of South Africa in early 2011 told of a reluctance to inform young people if they are HIV-positive for fear they might find the information "too traumatic." The ally of epidemiologists is an informed and responsible public. Blame who you will—the governments, the national media, education and health officials, the foreign NGOs—for such a long time, the message about HIV/AIDS and people's personal responsibilities for both themselves and those they were in contact with did not get out at anywhere near adequate levels.

Throughout Africa over thirty years, HIV/AIDS elicited a variety of responses. Because HIV/AIDS was so mysterious and people found it so frightening, they were willing to try almost anything and trust almost anybody. Every purveyor of magic potions or homeopathic remedies, every serious herbalist, and every scurrilous snake-oil salesman or witch doctor went to the cupboard to see what they could haul out. The disease turned out to be ripe for quackeries and fly-by-night cures built not on solid science, but (charitably) on hope or (not so charitably) on opportunism.

In the early 1990s, a drug called Kemron popped up in Kenya. It came out of a respectable lab, so caused particular problems. Dr Davey Koech, a highly placed relative of the Kenyan President Daniel Arap Moi, had been trained in the United States, at the University of Nevada. Back in Nairobi he had collaborated with the North Americans from his position as director of KEMRI, working hand in hand with some of the research projects conducting, for example, the CD4 counts for the sex workers studied by Joan Kreiss. For this, he was listed as a co-author in the ensuing publication in the *New England Journal of Medicine*. Out of the blue, though, Koech claimed he had developed a "cure" for AIDS. His partner was an American named Joseph Cummins who, back in Texas, had used low doses of alpha interferon to treat respiratory infections in cattle before trying it out on his mother-in-law's melanoma. When Cummins visited Kenya to undertake a cattle study, he met Koech, who became intrigued about the properties of interferon, wondering what its effect might be on people suffering from HIV/AIDS. Cummins started sending a new powdered form of the drug to Koech, who had his patients ingest a daily dose of it by eating it on wafers. He gave the product the trade name "Kemron," and within months declared the treatment a success. Published reports (co-authored by Cummins) claimed that ninety-nine out of 101 patients became outwardly healthy on the treatment. Their AIDS symptoms vanished, some regained huge numbers of immune cells, and some even stopped exhibiting HIV in their blood.

The findings on Kemron were far from definitive. Because no comparison had been made between treated and untreated patients, it was hard to know how much if any of the improvement the patients seemed to enjoy was due to the drug. But that didn't dampen the enthusiasm of the Kenyan government or its admirers elsewhere. At a rally marking the formal launch of Kemron, President Moi announced that fifty HIV/AIDS victims had already been cured. The *Nation* newspaper ran photographs of Koech holding up a vial of Kemron—about the size, Frank Plummer recalls, of the cap of a Bic pen—and bragging about the results. The Kenyan press, and some of the world media, touted "a cure for AIDS made in Africa." Before long, oral interferon was circulating in underground HIV/AIDS "buyers' clubs," and all kinds of people, including HIV-infected sex workers, were taking it.

Kemron was only one of many so-called treatments or cures. Over the decades, numerous would-be saviours popped up wanting to give the public hope—and walk away with money in their pockets. Cures were promised, relief was signalled to be at hand. The purveyors, who ran the gamut from crass opportunists to traditional medicine men, offered sometimes harmless homeopathic medicines, at other times their "cures" were outright dangerous. In 1996 in South Africa, something called DMF, or dimethylformamide, was created by a Pretoria-based medical technician named Olga Visser as a treatment for AIDS. Under the product name Virodene, it got as far as a human trial before it was denounced as a toxic chemical that could cause everything from skin rashes to liver damage. In 2003, South African government researchers were discovered in Tanzania treating HIV-positive people with something called oxihumate-K, a drug derived from garden fertilizer. In 1996, another Kenyan government scientist, Arthur Obel, came up with a concoction—both in liquid and powder form—he called Pearl Omega, which he claimed took away the symptoms of AIDS. The revolving door of purported magical cures created a difficult time for the Western scientists in Nairobi, who knew full well the treatments being so widely purveyed were bogus. As Allan Ronald put it, "We had to survive this total hocus-pocus. Sex workers were being treated with Kemron and we weren't allowed to say anything negative." Eventually, it all collapsed. In Kemron's case, the product was tested in a randomized trial funded by the WHO that debunked its curative properties. It was labelled a homeopathic medicine, so did no harm except that it persuaded people they had a cure when they had no such thing, and thus became a detour on the road. The other harm was that its connection to the office of the president meant that critics who deigned to speak out found themselves in trouble.

Behind all this, though, some observers noted a phenomenon that was possibly far more complicated than simple quackery or rank opportunism. At the

2006 International AIDS Conference held in Toronto, South Africa's health minister, Manto Tshabalala-Msimang, set up a public health display that focussed neither on antiretroviral drugs nor on preventive measures like condom distribution. Instead, she set out "natural" potions created out of beetroot, olive oil, garlic, lemons, and African potatoes with the message that HIV/AIDS could be combatted by ingesting these elixirs. To say this caused a "stir" is too kind. The main response from the hundreds of other officials, scientists, and activists, including Bill Clinton and Bill Gates, was outrage. Yet the collision was not something that had come out of the blue. At the very highest levels of the Ministry of Health and the office of the Director General of Health, offices with reach directly into the circle of President Thabo Mbeki himself, South Africa had for some time not only disdained but publicly attacked the prevailing scientific consensus on the cause and treatment of HIV/AIDS. The disease was caused not by a virus, they suggested, but by poverty, and the West's response to the African HIV/AIDS crisis was a form of scientific imperialism.

This set the scene for a tempestuous fight where the strategies of the Western HIV/AIDS organizations were thrown topsy-turvy. While South Africa's HIV rates continued to skyrocket, officials like Tshabalala-Msimang decried antiretroviral drugs as "toxic, damaging, and poisonous." It would have been easy to try to isolate a few individuals and label them irrational crackpots. But what was really going on appeared to be something much bigger, an attack, orchestrated at the highest levels, on science itself, or at least an opting out of science. This was impossible to explain, save through, perhaps, some reactive anti-Western prism that equated science and the scientific method with another colonial imposition. The creation of science or, as it was earlier and more broadly called, "natural history," Mary Louise Pratt declared in *Imperial Eyes*, "asserted an urban, lettered, male authority over the whole of the planet."[11] It was in that sense "Western," even though practised throughout the world. It came out of the Enlightenment and had unquestioned authority and power that it dared anyone to question.

What was South Africa doing? Were its officials total idiots, or was this a politico-cultural game with them employing the only means the non-Western world (according to Pratt's paradigm) had available in order to fight back? It was a ludicrously difficult fight to be sure, for in any argument against science the very discourse is owned by the other side. What's more, given the power of the orthodoxy science has come to possess, one could only suffer ridicule and become marginalized by going up against it. Yet the fact it was happening deserved examination that was more serious than simple disdain. What got labelled

AIDS denial was in reality a kind of supreme anti-Western gesture couched in the guise of anti-science. It might also have represented peoples' growing desperation around the unsolved puzzle of HIV/AIDS and the inability of even the discipline of science to slay it.

President Thabo Mbeki was, arguably, half right. He was universally decried as wrong on the virus statement—AIDS is caused by the HIV virus—but the epidemic created by the virus might well have been perpetuated by poverty. That is certainly what tracking numbers identifying the communities of the world affected by the epidemic—and all other infectious disease epidemics—suggest. At the end of the twentieth century, infectious diseases accounted for less than 5 percent of serious morbidity and deaths in industrialized countries, yet caused one-third of all deaths in the developing world. Of all things that separate these two halves of our world, the disparities around rampaging infectious diseases is the biggest. The imbalance, furthermore, persists in the allotment of resources. More than 90 percent of preventable mortality from infectious diseases occurs in the developing world, yet only 5 percent of global health research dollars target the health problems of those countries.[12] On the basis of these numbers, almost all infectious diseases specialists can understand that the calling to work in their field incorporates a call to both social and economic justice.

When we think about innovations that have changed the world, that have been the true revolutions in human health—and mean that we live longer and have better quality lives with less suffering and less pain, and feel greater pleasure and well-being when we do live—two things come to mind: public sanitation and control of infectious diseases. The fundamentals of both are considered to be of public rather than private health because their beneficiaries are the entirety of the community. In the long-run, who can say whether germs and viruses might still win out in some final battle? But in the much shorter story of human medical history, both have seen moments of attack from the honourable armies of public health. The ensuing setbacks for viruses and germs have changed human history and human existence.

The search for interventions continues to turn up discoveries or creations that cause flurries of excitement. In the summer of 2010, just in time for the eighteenth International AIDS Conference, this time in Vienna, scientists from South Africa introduced what they called the "invisible condom." A vaginal microbicide gel that could be used by a woman without her male sex partner knowing was heralded as "the best AIDS-prevention news in years."[13] By skirting the thorny issue of male resistance to wearing condoms, it would also place power and control into the hands of women. The protection rate in trials in South Africa was 39 percent. This, admittedly, was not high, but the product with at least a limited rate of proven success followed a dozen attempts at producing such a microbicide that were all total failures. And it was touted as being available for two cents a dose, although the applicator costs forty cents. AIDS, however, certainly in Africa, remains a war that is far from won.

The president of the International AIDS Society is Julio Montaner, an Argentinean-born Canadian who came to prominence as a medical doctor and advocate for Vancouver's safe injection site for intravenous drug users. His take on the future underlines the stark dichotomy of HIV/AIDS. "While entirely preventable," he says, "it continues to spread. And there is no cure." For the countries dealing with it, the challenge remains monumental, as is the dilemma about what long-term actions are truly doable. The population of Kenya in 2010 is over 38 million, and 1.4 million have AIDS. Forty percent of them receive antiretroviral therapies. In the population of those between the ages of fifteen and sixty-four, the active sexual years, 7.2 percent of Kenyans are HIV-positive; in Nyanza province in western Kenya, the number is doubled to 14.9 percent. Each year 90,000 Kenyans die of AIDS; meanwhile there are 140,000 new infections. Sixty percent of government health spending in Kenya goes toward AIDS, leaving 40 percent for all other diseases. Yet 98 percent of HIV/AIDS work in Kenya is financed by foreign donors. "How is this sustainable?" asks Omu Anzala, the Canadian-trained chair of his country's medical school microbiology department.

"Targeting interventions towards high-risk groups, which we know has a huge impact on HIV transmission, is still not fully accepted," remains Frank Plummer's contention. It is a sobering final statement with which to close this examination of Africa's devastating HIV/AIDS epidemic. In a 2002 interview with the *Winnipeg Free Press*, Plummer called HIV/AIDS "now the greatest plague in human history," and added that the epidemic was the result of "a global failure of governments to do something about the spread of the fatal disease."[14] Eight years later I ask him if anything has changed. "This disease could have been prevented," he says yet again. "We knew how to do it. We were fighting a losing battle when we said, look, there are simple ways of preventing this. If the world had done what we knew in 1988, or in 1998, we would not have the problem we have now."

Afterword

BY KING HOLMES, HERBERT NSANZE,
PETER PIOT, AND ALLAN RONALD

S exually transmitted infections (STIs) were not a priority health issue in most developing countries in 1978. However, Herbert Nsanze, then Professor of Medical Microbiology at the University of Nairobi, was concerned about an epidemic of genital ulcer disease (GUD) being experienced at that time in Nairobi. Hundreds of men were queuing each day for care at the only STI clinic in Kenya, many with genital ulcers, and chancroid seemed the most likely diagnosis. George Antel from the World Health Organization connected Herbert to Allan Ronald at the University of Manitoba. The expertise gained in Winnipeg during the previous three years, following a chancroid outbreak in 1975, perhaps could help define and ultimately limit this painful, although at that time relatively unimportant ulcerating genital infection.

At that time, the burden of STIs in Kenya was largely unknown, HIV had not yet been recognized, and other infectious diseases were the focus of limited global collaboration. With a few outstanding exceptions, Western universities and governments were not allocating significant resources to academic activities in developing countries. However, the global eradication of smallpox in 1977 had provided a template for countries to collaborate successfully.

The University of Nairobi Collaborating Centre for STI research and training was established in 1980. We had no strategic plan, no specific goals, and no road map. We were young, enthusiastic, and committed to good science as a partial answer to the human dilemma of ill health. GUD, ophthalmia neonatorum, and pelvic inflammatory infections were our initial focus of work, and research in each area led to important discoveries and publications.

Cordial relations with African colleagues as well as with colleagues from the United States and Belgium enabled further success. In Kenya, the chairs of the Department of Medical Microbiology and the deans of the School of Medicine at the University of Nairobi have, over thirty years, been extremely supportive. In particular, we honour the memories of professors Hannington Pamba, Jack Ndinya-Achola, and Job Bwayo, all past chairs of the department. Challenges faced included jurisdiction, finances, communications, publication rights, and day-to-day responsibilities. Our success at dispute resolution and our shared commitment to science created the foundation on which we were able to build a long-term investment of fiscal and intellectual resources. In retrospect, our success also depended on at least two additional factors.

First, from the outset, we were successful in convincing some of our brightest trainees in Belgium, Canada, and the United States to spend several years with Kenyan colleagues co-leading research efforts. In an era before the Internet, connectivity was difficult, but was somehow achieved in order to support and enable relatively junior individuals to have adequate scientific and personal support. Young scientists such as Frank Plummer (Winnipeg), Joan Kreiss (Seattle), Marleen Temmerman (Antwerp), Stephen Moses (Winnipeg), and other fellows and junior faculty members were willing to live in Nairobi and assume scientific leadership alongside Kenyan colleagues. Individuals at multiple levels, from technologists and medical students through to residents, fellows, and faculty colleagues, came to Nairobi for shorter periods, and many Kenyans received travel fellowships for training in Western countries. We have identified over 300 individuals who have used this opportunity to contribute to the science, learn from each other, and experience different cultures. For most participants, these opportunities have had enduring impact on their personal and professional lives.

The second factor ensuring our success was the recognition in 1983 that the "new disease" AIDS was causing illness and death in Kenya. Studies by Joan Kreiss, Frank Plummer, Peter Piot, King Holmes, and others demonstrated that HIV was rapidly spreading in vulnerable populations, and in the general population. This created a momentum which continues today. The epidemic had to be urgently addressed, and in addition to strong prevention and care programs, this also required excellent science. In Africa, routes and dynamics of HIV transmission had to be determined, interventions to slow transmission implemented, and ultimately treatment issues addressed. Throughout, due to the scientific leadership within Kenya, and with substantial external funding support, resources were found to carry out definitive studies that have resulted in over 300 publications. The spirit of collaboration across all of the universities and other institutions involved, and a national commitment to problem solving through science, was productive and gratifying.

Throughout the past three decades, almost all program resources have come from specific projects funded largely by granting agencies that initially had a limited understanding of the costs and complexities of research in developing country settings. This caused many challenges to financial management, and for the best use of resources to achieve project objectives. However, many individuals used their leadership positions at their universities in Canada, the United States, and Belgium to ensure that planning and sharing occurred, and financial resources were optimized.

From the onset, the collaboration in Kenya intended that evidence derived from well-conducted research would be implemented within the Kenyan health care system. Usually this occurred through influencing decision makers within the Ministry of Health, training individuals who would become leaders within the university and government structures, publishing articles in high-impact journals (including success stories), and holding an annual scientific retreat. The Government of Canada, through the Canadian International Development Agency (CIDA), for almost two decades supported sexually transmitted infection and HIV prevention and control programs in Kenya under the leadership of Drs. Elizabeth Ngugi and Stephen Moses. Knowledge acquired about the contribution of chancroid and other STIs to the spread of HIV has enhanced the value of these programs, reducing substantially HIV transmission. Chancroid, the STI that started the collaborative venture, has now been eliminated from Kenya, with no proven cases since 1999.

Funding for capital infrastructure has always been extremely difficult to obtain. Fortunately, several patrons donated funds for an initial laboratory facility, and in 2005 the Canadian Foundation for Innovation provided $3.3 million to build a Microbiology Research Centre at the University of Nairobi, which will take us well into the future.

What does the future hold? We remain confident that the young Kenyans and their global partners who have acquired leadership and managerial skills, as well as a sound scientific foundation, will continue the collaborative work for many years. Our hope is that more funding will become available in Kenya for good science, as well as more opportunities for funding from Western sources. We are enthusiastic about ongoing linkages with other African research sites, and with increasing scientific interdependence within Africa. We also believe that there will be ongoing mutual and reciprocal benefits from scientific collaboration between Kenya and Western countries. We need each other. Science rapidly evolves with new ideas and technologies. Their introduction into Kenya and other African countries is essential for academic excellence, and for the creation of capacity for robust local problem solving.

In conclusion, the four of us are extremely grateful to the University of Nairobi, the Government of Kenya, the Kenya Medical Research Institute, and the hundreds of colleagues who have facilitated our shared endeavours. Kenya and Kenyans have made a substantial contribution to our growth as individuals, and to our shared enterprise of using science as a major strategy for development.

Finally, our thanks to Larry Krotz who carried out the field research for, and then wrote, this book that has become the story of our endeavour. We hope that it may influence others who share our goals to partner with colleagues in contexts of limited resources to improve health through the "academic enterprise" of generating, exchanging, translating, and using knowledge. We also sincerely thank the University of Manitoba and the Winnipeg Foundation for their moral and financial support over many decades. We hope you enjoyed the story!

King Holmes
Herbert Nsanze
Peter Piot
Allan Ronald

Selected Bibliography

Beck, Edward, Nicholas Mays, Alan Whiteside, and Jose Zuniga. *The HIV Pandemic: Local and Global Implications*. Oxford: Oxford University Press, 2006.

Caldwell, John C., and Pat Caldwell. "The African AIDS Epidemic." *Scientific American*, March 1996.

Campbell, Catherine. *Letting Them Die: Why HIV/AIDS Prevention Programmes Fail*. Bloomington: Indiana University Press, 2003.

Chin, James. *The AIDS Pandemic: The Collision of Epidemiology with Political Correctness*. Oxford: Radcliffe Publishing, 2007.

Conover, Ted. "Trucking Through the AIDS Belt." *New Yorker*, August 16, 1993.

Crawford, Dorothy. *Deadly Companions: How Microbes Shaped our History*. New York: Oxford University Press, 2007.

Engel, Jonathan. *The Epidemic: A Global History of AIDS*. New York: Harper Collins, 2006.

Epstein, Helen. *The Invisible Cure: Africa, the West, and the Fight against AIDS*. New York: Farrar, Straus, Giroux, 2007.

Fox, Donald, and Elizabeth Fee, eds. *AIDS: The Making of a Chronic Disease*. Berkeley: University of California Press, 1992.

Garrett, Laurie. *Betrayal of Trust: The Collapse of Global Public Health*. New York: Hyperion, 2000.

Hooper, Edward. *The River: A Journey to the Source of HIV and AIDS*. Boston: Little Brown, 1999.

Hunter, Susan. *Black Death: AIDS in Africa*. New York: Palgrave Macmillan, 2003.

Illiffe, John. *The African AIDS Epidemic: A History*. Athens, OH: Ohio University Press, 2006.

Itano, Nicole. *No Place to Bury the Dead: Denial, Despair and Hope in the African AIDS Pandemic*. New York: Simon and Shuster, 2007.

Kalipeni, Ezekiel. *Strong Women, Dangerous Times: Gender and HIV/AIDS in Africa*. New York: Nova Science Publishers, 2009.

Kalipeni, Ezekial, Susan Craddock, Josgh Oppong, and Jayata Ghosh. *HIV and AIDS in Africa: Beyond Epidemiology*. Hoboken, NJ: Wiley-Blackwell, 2003.

Kidder, Tracy. *Mountains Beyond Mountains: The Quest of Dr. Paul Farmer, A Man who would Cure the World*. New York: Random House, 2003.

Lewis, Stephen. *Race Against Time: Searching for Hope in AIDS-Ravaged Africa*. Toronto: Anansi, 2006.

Mukudi, Edith, and Stephen Commins. *HIV/AIDS in Africa*. Trenton, NJ: Africa World Press, 2008.

Nolen, Stephanie. *28 Stories of AIDS in Africa*. Toronto: Knopf Canada, 2007.

Nowak, Rachel. "Staging Ethical AIDS Trials in Africa." *Science*, September 8, 1995.

Oldstone, Michael. *Viruses, Plagues and History*. New York: Oxford University Press, 2010.

Packard, Randall M., and Paul Epstein. "Medical Research on AIDS in Africa, a Historical Perspective." In *AIDS: The Making of a Chronic Disease*, ed. Donald Fox and Elizabeth Fee. Berkeley: University of California Press, 1992.

Pepin, Jacques. *The Origin of AIDS*, Cambridge: Cambridge University Press, 2011.

Pisani, Elizabeth. *The Wisdom of Whores: Bureaucrats, Brothels, and the Business of AIDS*. Toronto: Viking Penguin, 2008.

Poku, Nana K. *AIDS in Africa: How The Poor Are Dying*. Cambridge: Polity Press, 2005.

Pratt, Mary Louise. *Imperial Eyes: Travel Writing and Transculturation*. New York: Routledge, 1992.

Ronald, Allan. "The Nairobi STD Program: An International Partnership." *Infectious Disease Clinics of North America* 5, 2 (1991): 337–52.

Smith, Michael. "Partners in a Pandemic." *University Affairs*, April 11, 2005.

Sontag, Susan. *AIDS and Its Metaphors*. New York: Farrar, Straus and Giroux, 1988.

Treichler, Paula. "AIDS and HIV Infection in the Third World." In *AIDS: The Making of a Chronic Disease*, ed. Fox and Fee.

UNAIDS. *2006 Report on the Global AIDS Epidemic: 10th Anniversary Special Edition*. Geneva: UNAIDS, 2006. http://data.unAIDS.org/Publications/IRC-pub07/jc1238-execsumglobrep_en.pdf.

World Bank. *Intensifying Action Against HIV AIDS in Africa: Responding to a Developmental Crisis*. Washington, DC: World Bank, 1999. http://siteresources.worldbank.org/AFRICAEXT/Resources/AIDStrat.pdf.

——. *The World Bank's Commitment to HIV AIDS in Africa: Our Agenda for Action*. Washington, DC: World Bank, 2008. http://siteresources.worldbank.org/EXTAFRREGTOPHIVAIDS/Resources/AFA_Brochure.pdf.

Notes

INTRODUCTION

1   Susan Sontag, *AIDS and Its Metaphors* (New York: Farrar, Straus and Giroux, 1988), 82.

2   The project known as UNIM—for the universities of Nairobi, Illinois, and Manitoba—was one of three clinical trials going on simultaneously between 2002 and 2007; the other two were conducted in Uganda and South Africa. All three reached the same conclusions and all were stopped early due to the overwhelming power of their statistics.

3   Sharif R. Sawires, Shari L. Dworkin, Agnès Fiamma, Dean Peacock, Greg Szekeres, and Thomas J Coates, "Male Circumcision and HIV/AIDS: Challenges and Opportunities," *Lancet* 369, 9562 (February 24, 2007): 708.

4   Over the course of those years I published articles in various Canadian publications including *Maclean's*, the *Walrus*, the *United Church Observer*, the University of Manitoba *Alumni Journal*, and the *National Post* newspaper. I also wrote and directed a film for the National Film Board of Canada (1998), titled *Searching for Hawa's Secret*.

5   Elizabeth Pisani, *The Wisdom of Whores; Bureaucrats, Brothels, and the Business of AIDS*. (Toronto: Viking Penguin, 2008), 5.

6   One important recent history of AIDS is Jacques Pepin's *The Origin of AIDS* (Cambridge: Cambridge University Press, 2011).

7   According to former UNAIDS chief Peter Piot, 1.3 million people (72 percent of all AIDS deaths) died of the disease in sub-Saharan Africa in 2009.

8   Statistics from *UNAIDS Report on the Global AIDS Epidemic, 2010*, http://www.unAIDS.org/globalreport/global_report.htm.

9   The following are journal articles by scientists from the Nairobi collaboration relating to the potential role of circumcision published a full decade before it gained broad recognition as a viable strategy: D.W. Cameron, J.N. Simonsen, L.J. D'Costa, G.M. Maitha, M. Gakinya, M. Cheang, J.O. Ndinya-Achola, P. Piot, R.C. Brunham, A.R. Ronald, and F.A. Plummer, "Female to Male Transmission of Human Immunodeficiency Virus Type 1: Risk Factors for Seroconversion in Men," *Lancet* 334, 8660 (1989): 403–7; J.N. Simonsen, D.W. Cameron, M.N. Gakinya, J.O. Ndinya-Achola, L.J. D'Costa, P. Karasira, M. Cheang, A.R. Ronald, P. Piot, and F.A. Plummer, "Human Immunodeficiency Virus Infection Among Men with Sexually Transmitted Diseases. Experience from a Center in Africa," *New England Journal of Medicine* 319 (1988): 274–8; S. Moses, J.E. Bradley, N.J.D. Nagelkerke, J.O. Ndinya-Achola, A.R. Ronald, and F.A. Plummer, "Geographical Patterns of Male Circumcision Practices in Africa: Association with HIV Prevalence," *International Journal of Epidemiology* 19, 3 (1990):

693–97. Many of the same authors dealt with the matter again in the body of another article: A.R. Ronald, F.A. Plummer, E. Ngugi, J.O. Ndinya-Achola, P. Piot, J. Kreiss, and R. Brunham, "The Nairobi STD Program: An International Partnership," *Infectious Disease Clinics of North America* 5, 2 (1991): 337–52.

10 Helen Epstein, *The Invisible Cure: Africa, the West, and the Fight against AIDS* (New York: Farrar, Straus, and Giroux, 2007), 266.

CHAPTER 1: WAGING WAR WITH INFECTIOUS DISEASES

1 Y. Al-Mazrou, S. Berkley, B. Bloom, et al., "A Vital Opportunity for Global Health," *Lancet* 350, 9080 (1997): 750–1.

2 Dorothy Crawford, *Deadly Companions: How Microbes Shaped our History* (Oxford: Oxford University Press, 2007), 12.

3 Quoted in Michael Oldstone, *Viruses, Plagues and History* (New York: Oxford University Press, 2010), 10.

4 Ibid., 268.

5 Louis Pasteur was the father of pasteurization, the process to kill bacteria; Koch isolated tuberculosis bacillus and cholera vibrio bacteria in the 1880s.

6 Crawford, *Deadly Companions*, 184.

7 Ibid., 188.

8 J.M. Bumsted, *The University of Manitoba: An Illustrated History* (Winnipeg: University of Manitoba Press, 2001), 8.

9 Ibid., 80.

10 The Canadian Medical Research Council (now CIHR, the Canadian Institutes of Health Research) was created in 1960. Friesen was president from 1991 to 1999 and helped transform the organization into the CIHR.

11 Bumsted, *Manitoba*, 175.

12 Honours bestowed on Ronald by the University of Manitoba include being named a distinguished professor of medicine; being recipient of a distinguished alumni award in 1990; and being inducted to the Canadian Medical Hall of Fame in 2010.

13 Crawford, *Deadly Companions*, 189.

14 On the Kenyan side of the collaboration, heads of the University of Nairobi department of medical microbiology were always the main link. Nsanze was followed by Professor Hannington Pamba, who served in that role between 1983 and 1987. (Years later, Pamba jovially talked about "the Canadian taxpayers, that mass of good-willed citizens without whom our clinics wouldn't be functioning.") He, in turn, was succeeded by Professor Isaac Wamola from 1987 to 1990, and followed by Dr Ndinya-Achola, Dr Job Bwayo, Dr Walter Jaoko, and Dr Omu Anzala.

CHAPTER 2: THE AFRICAN EPIDEMIC

1 Researchers who had visited Central Africa in late 1983 identified twenty-six patients with AIDS in Kigali, Rwanda, and thirty-eight in Kinshasa, Zaire. The Rwandan study concluded that "an association of an urban environment, a relatively high income, and heterosexual promiscuity could be a risk factor for AIDS in Africa." Philippe Van De Perre, et al., "Acquired Immunodeficiency Syndrome in Rwanda," *Lancet* 324, 8394 (1984): 62–65.

2 Joan Kreiss, telephone and e-mail interview, May 2010.

3   To gather personal recollections about this highly charged time in Kenya, I interviewed Frank Plummer, Leslie Slaney, Peter Piot, Larry Gelmon (who by 2010 was working for the project and had been resident in Nairobi since 1993), Joanne Embree, King Holmes, Allan Ronald, Stephen Moses, and Elizabeth Ngugi.

4   Epstein, *Invisible Cure*, 155.

5   Ibid., 161. The term for AIDS in Swahili is *Ukimwe*, which means "slim."

6   Oldstone, *Viruses, Plagues and History*, 264–6.

7   Stephen Pincock, "HIV Discoverers Awarded Nobel Prize for Medicine," *Lancet* 372, 9647 (2008): 1373.

8   Richard Horton and Pam Das, "Putting Prevention at the Forefront of HIV/AIDS," *Lancet* 372, 9637 (2008): 421.

9   Paula Treichler, "AIDS and HIV Infection in the Third World," in *AIDS: The Making of a Chronic Disease*, ed. Donald Fox and Elizabeth Fee (Berkeley: University of California Press, 1992), 391.

10   Pisani, *Wisdom of Whores*, 134.

11   John Caldwell and Pat Caldwell, "The African AIDS Epidemic," *Scientific American*, March 1996, 62.

12   Ibid.

13   Randall M. Packard and Paul Epstein, "Medical Research on AIDS in Africa, a Historical Perspective," in *AIDS: The Making of a Chronic Disease*, ed. Fox and Fee, 351–352.

14   Epstein, *Invisible Cure*, 49.

15   Population Research Institute, Pennsylvania State University, 2000.

16   Epstein, *Invisible Cure*, 60.

17   Caldwell and Caldwell, "African AIDS Epidemic," 66.

18   Data to support this was analyzed by Daniel Halperin, a medical anthropologist working for USAID's Global Health Program.

19   Ted Conover, "Trucking Through the AIDS Belt," *New Yorker*, August 16, 1993.

20   Bwayo would later serve as chair of microbiology at the University of Nairobi. His research with truck drivers was funded by the University of Washington and the University of Manitoba. The research was published: J. Bwayo, F. Plummer, M. Omari, A. Mutere, S. Moses, J. Ndinya-Achola, P. Velentgas, and J. Kreiss, "Human Immunodeficiency Virus Infection in Long-Distance Truck Drivers in East Africa," *Archives of Internal Medicine* 154 (1994): 1391–6.

21   J.K. Kreiss, D. Koech, F.A. Plummer, K.K. Holmes, M. Lightfoote, P. Piot, A.R. Ronald, J.O. Ndinya-Achola, L.J. D'Costa, P. Roberts, E.N. Ngugi, and T.C. Quinn, "AIDS Virus Infection in Nairobi Prostitutes: Extension of the Epidemic to East Africa," *New England Journal of Medicine* 314 (1986): 414–8.

22   Lawrence Altman, "AIDS in Africa a Pattern of Mystery," *New York Times*, November 8, 1985.

23   Lawrence K. Altman, "Linking AIDS to Africa Provokes Bitter Debate," *New York Times*, November 21, 1985.

24   Sontag, *AIDS and Its Metaphors*, 27.

25   J.N. Simonsen, F.A. Plummer, E.N. Ngugi, C. Black, J. Kreiss, M.N. Gakinya, P. Waiyaki, G. Vercauteren, L. Slaney, J. Koss, L.J. D'Costa, J.O. Ndinya-Achola, P. Karasira, J. Kimata, P. Piot, M. Cheang, and A.R. Ronald, "HIV Infection among Lower Socioeconomic Strata Prostitutes in Nairobi," *AIDS* 4 (1990): 139–44.

CHAPTER 3: EDUCATING AROUND AIDS

1   USAID sources claim $7 billion as their expenditure on AIDS up to 2011.

2   Robert Cushman, "The Kenyan National AIDS Control Programme and Strategies for CIDA's Involvement," Consultant's Report, March 15, 1989.

3   Letter from Robert Cushman to Allan Ronald, April 4, 1989.

4   My young friend might have done well to look up the top ten causes of death among persons aged fifteen to fifty-nine, according to the Global Burden of Disease study (2001):

      1. HIV/AIDS, 13.2%

      2. Ischemic heart disease, 8.3%

      3. Tuberculosis, 6.6%

      4. Road Traffic deaths, 5.2%

      5. Cerebral vascular disease, 4.9%

      6. Self inflicted injuries, 4.3%

      7. Violence, 3%

      8. Cirrhosis of liver, 2.4%

      9. Lower respiratory disease, 2.2%

      10. Chronic obstructive pulmonary disease, 2.1%

See James Chin, *The AIDS Pandemic: The Collision of Epidemiology with Political Correctness* (Oxford: Radcliffe Publishing, 2007), 184.

5   Gerri Dickson, "Strengthening STD/AIDS Control in Kenya," Kenya STD/AIDS Control Project, Monitoring Report No. 2, July 5, 1992.

6   Stephen Moses, "Strengthening STD/AIDS Control in Kenya," Quarterly Progress Report No. 7, October 16, 1992.

7   In 1996, Moses left the position of director. He was followed by a series of others; the three following were Denis Jackson, Aine Costigan, and Chester Morris. The project was well-enough-regarded that its funder, CIDA, agreed to copy it, setting up, in 1997, a program to take the lessons of Kenya beyond Kenyan borders. Directed by Larry Gelmon, the Regional AIDS Training Network (RATN) set out to initiate HIV training in eleven countries—Kenya, Uganda, Rwanda, Tanzania, Zimbabwe, Zambia, Malawi, Lesotho, Botswana, Swaziland, and the Republic of South Africa.

8   CIDA-funded projects in West Africa attached to the Laval University, and SARDC, the Southern Africa Regional Development Center in Zimbabwe, both closed their doors at that time.

CHAPTER 4: RESEARCH STRATEGIES

1   Peter Karasira was trained at Makerere University in his home country of Uganda, but had left there, chased out by the violence of Idi Amin and Milton Obote. He went to Nairobi where he got a job in the university's department of medical microbiology. He worked with Margaret Fast and Joan Kreiss. In 1985, Neil Simonsen remembers befriending Karasira and the two of them travelling to Kampala and then to Karasira's hometown of Jinja, where the Nile joins Lake Victoria. There they visited Karasira's wife, parents, and four children. They had a delightful time, says Simonsen, before returning to Nairobi. A short while later, Peter began to complain of feeling unwell. He discovered that he was HIV-positive, though for a long time he did not discuss it with anybody. This was a time when even Kenyans who knew a lot about AIDS and worked with it in the scientific community were highly aware of being stigmatized. Karasira maintained

his secret for two years, until the first symptoms of an AIDS-defining illness appeared. In the early 1990s, Peter Karasira, then in his early forties, died.

2   P. Piot, F.A. Plummer, M.-A. Rey, E.N. Ngugi, C. Rouzioux, J.O. Ndinya-Achola, G. Vercauteren, L.J. D'Costa, M. Laga, H. Nsanze, L. Fransen, D. Haase, G. van der Groen, R.C. Brunham, A.R. Ronald, and F. Brun-Vezinet, "Retrospective Seroepidemiology of AIDS Virus Infection in Nairobi Populations," *Journal of Infectious Diseases* 155 (1987): 1108–12.

3   J.N. Simonsen, D.W. Cameron, M.N. Gakinya, J.O. Ndinya-Achola, L.J. D'Costa, P. Karasira, M. Cheang, A.R. Ronald, P. Piot, and F.A. Plummer, "Human Immunodeficiency Virus Infection among Men with Sexually Transmitted Diseases. Experience from a Center in Africa," *New England Journal of Medicine* 319 (1988): 274–8; E.N. Ngugi, F.A. Plummer, J.N. Simonsen, D.W. Cameron, M. Bosire, P. Waiyaki, A.R. Ronald, and J.O. Ndinya-Achola, "Prevention of Transmission of Human Immunodefieny Virus in Africa: Effectiveness of Condom Promotion and Health Education among Prostitutes," *Lancet* 332, 8616 (1988): 887–90.

4   A table compiled by Frank Plummer and Mark Tyndall, referenced in Jonathan Engel, *The Epidemic, A Global History of AIDS* (New York: Smithsonian Books, 2006), neatly summarizes the infection patterns of Nairobi men who frequented prostitutes: 2.5 percent of circumcised men with no genital ulcer disease (GUD) tested HIV-positive; 13.4 percent of circumcised men *with* GUDs were HIV-positive; and uncircumcised men with no GUDs proved 29 percent HIV-positive, a number that rose to an appalling 53 percent for those at the far end of the scale, not circumcised and possessing genital ulcers.

5   J.N. Simonsen, F.A. Plummer, E.N. Ngugi, C. Black, J. Kreiss, M.N. Gakinya, P. Waiyaki, G. Vercauteren, L. Slaney, J. Koss, L.J. D'Costa, J.O. Ndinya-Achola, P. Karasira, J. Kimata, P. Piot, M. Cheang, and A.R. Ronald, "HIV Infection among Lower Socioeconomic Strata Prostitutes in Nairobi," *AIDS* 4, 2 (1990): 139–44.

6   Michele Barry, "Ethical Considerations of Human Investigation in Developing Countries. The AIDS Dilemma," *New England Journal of Medicine* 319, 16 (1988): 1083–6.

7   Ibid., 1083.

8   Ibid., 1084.

9   Ibid.

10   Tetracycline cream will work just as well.

11   Oldstone, *Viruses, Plagues and History*, 274.

12   P. Datta, J.E. Embree, J.K. Kreiss, J.O. Ndinya-Achola, M. Braddick, M. Temmerman, N.J.D. Nagelkerke, G. Maitha, K.K. Holmes, P. Piot, H.O. Pamba, and F.A. Plummer, "Mother to Child Transmission of Human Immunodeficiency Virus Type 1: Report from the Nairobi study," *Journal of Infectious Diseases* 170 (1994): 1134–40.

13   Now, with antiretroviral therapies, this is happily no longer the case. It looks as though HIV-positive mothers can continue to breast-feed if they are on antiretroviral therapies. This is the best of both worlds, allowing the many health advantages of breast-feeding without the risk of HIV transmission.

14   P. Datta, J.E. Embree, J.K. Kreiss, J.O. Ndinya-Achola, J. Muriithi, K.K. Holmes, and F.A. Plummer, "Resumption of Breast-feeding in Later Childhood. A Risk Factor for Mother to Child Human Immunodeficiency Virus Type 1 Transmission," *Pediatric Infectious Diseases Journal* 19 (1992): 309–14.

15   N.J.D. Nagelkerke, S. Moses, J.E. Embree, F. Jenniskens, and F.A. Plummer, "The Duration of Breast-feeding by HIV-1 Infected Mothers in Developing Countries:

Balancing benefits and risks," *Journal of Acquired Immune Deficiency Syndromes and Human Retrovirology* 8 (1995): 176–81.

16   Funds were provided by the Winnipeg Foundation, the Winnipeg-based Richardson Foundation, and a private donor, the Murphy family.

17   Interview with King Holmes, Nairobi, January 2010. King Holmes believes that in terms of physical infrastructure, they were, in fact, weaker than the Canadians, and credits his northern neighbours with carrying the ball on that aspect. "NIH federal funding precluded bricks and mortar," Holmes says.

18   J.N. Simonsen, D.W. Cameron, M.N. Gakinya, J.O. Ndinya-Achola, L.J. D'Costa, P. Karasira, M. Cheang, A.R. Ronald, P. Piot, and F.A. Plummer, "Human Immunodeficiency Virus Infection among Men with Sexually Transmitted Diseases. Experience from a center in Africa," *New England Journal of Medicine* 319 (1988): 274–8.

CHAPTER 5: SECRETS OF THE SEX WORKERS

1   K.R. Fowke, N.J.D. Nagelkerke, J. Kimani, J.N. Simonsen, A.O. Anzala, J.J. Bwayo, K.S. MacDonald, E.N. Ngugi, and F.A. Plummer, "Resistance to HIV-1 Infection among Persistently Seronegative Prostitutes in Nairobi, Kenya," *Lancet* 348, 9038 (1996): 1347–51.

2   Ian Maclean, interview with the author, 2010.

3   Avenue Flats, walking distance to Kenyatta National Hospital and the University of Nairobi medical school, provided apartments for a revolving door of Canadian, American and European researchers connected to the collaboration. Like almost all residential compounds in Nairobi, it was gated and had its own guards or *askaris*.

CHAPTER 6: THE VACCINE QUEST; AND MORE LESSONS FROM THE IMMUNE SYSTEM

1   The Government of Canada, supportive of IAVI, still set up its own program, CHVI, the Canadian HIV Vaccine Initiative, a decade later, in 2007.

2   Sarah Rowland-Jones, interview with the author, Oxford, U.K., June 2010.

3   S.L. Rowland-Jones, T. Dong, K.R. Fowke, J. Kimani, P. Krausa, H. Newell, T. Blanchard, K. Ariyoshi, J. Oyugi, E. Ngugi, J. Bwayo, K.S. MacDonald, A.J. McMichael, and F.A. Plummer, "Cytotoxic T-cell Responses to Multiple Conserved HIV Epitopes in HIV-Resistant Prostitutes in Nairobi," *Journal of Clinical Investigation* 102 (1998): 1758–65.

4   One was Rupert Kaul, who now became a doctoral student co-supervised by Rowland-Jones and Frank Plummer. There were also two Kenyans, Dr Omu Anzala and Dr Walter Jaoko. Jaoko, who would become chair of medical microbiology at the University of Nairobi in 2002, already had a D.Phil. from Oxford. His friend, Anzala, who like Jaoko had received his medical training in Nairobi (after which he worked as the second of the series of on-site clinicians at the Majengo clinic before leaving to get his PhD in Winnipeg), had gone to Oxford on a post-doctoral fellowship from 1996 to 1999. While there, his supervisor had been Rowland-Jones. They all settled in with the single purpose of getting the vaccine initiative underway. Heading up the entire team was Oxford professor Dr Andrew McMichael (now Sir Andrew McMichael FRS, a top-level immunologist who had been working on T cell immune responses to virus infections since 1977).

5   Jeff Otieno, *Daily Nation* (Nairobi), January 4, 2001.

6   Ibid.

7   Drs Anzala and Jaoko were interviewed by the author in Nairobi in January 2010.

8   R. Kaul, S.L. Rowland-Jones, J. Kimani, T. Dong, H.-B. Yang, P. Kiama, T. Rostron, E. Njagi, J.J. Bwayo, K.S. MacDonald, A.J. McMichael, and F.A. Plummer, "Late Seroconversion in HIV-Resistant Nairobi Prostitutes Despite Pre-existing HIV-specific CD8(+) Responses," *Journal of Clinical Investigation* 107 (2001): 341–9.

9   Following are some of the articles resulting from research in these areas: R. Kaul, J. Kimani, N. Nagelkerke, K. Fonck, E. Ngugi, F. Keli, K.S. MacDonald, I.W. Maclean, J.J. Bwayo, M. Temmerman, A.R. Ronald, and S. Moses, "Monthly antibiotic chemoprophylaxis and incidence of sexually transmitted infections and HIV-1 infection in Kenyan sex workers: A randomized controlled trial," *Journal of the American Medical Association* 291 (2004): 2555–62; A. Rebbapragada, C. Wachihi, C. Pettengell, S. Sunderji, S. Huibner, W. Jaoko, B. Ball, K. Fowke, T. Mazzulli, F.A. Plummer, and R. Kaul, "Negative mucosal synergy between Herpes simplex type 2 and HIV in the female genital tract," *AIDS* 21 (2007): 589–98; R. Kaul, D. Trabattoni, J.J. Bwayo, D. Arienti, A. Zagliani, F. Mwangi, E. Ngugi, K.S. MacDonald, T.B. Ball, M. Clerici, and F.A. Plummer, "HIV-1 specific mucosal IgA in a cohort of highly-exposed, HIV-1 sero-negative Kenyan prostitutes," *AIDS* 13 (1999): 23–9; R. Kaul, F.A. Plummer, J. Kimani, T. Dong, P. Kiama, T. Rostron, E. Njagi, K.S. MacDonald, J.J. Bwayo, A.J. McMichael, S.L. Rowland-Jones, "HIV-1 specific mucosal CD8+ lymphocyte responses in the cervix of HIV-1 resistant prostitutes in Nairobi," *Journal of Immunology* 164 (2000): 1602–11; R. Kaul, T. Dong, F.A. Plummer, J. Kimani, T. Rostron, P. Kiama, E. Njagi, E. Irungu, B. Farah, J. Oyugi, R. Chakraborty, K.S. MacDonald, J.J. Bwayo, A.J. McMichael, and S.L. Rowland-Jones, "CD8+ lymphocytes respond to different HIV epitopes in sero-negative and infected subjects," *Journal of Clinical Investigation* 107 (2001): 1303–10.

10   Graeme Smith, "The Bug Hunter of Winnipeg," *Globe and Mail*, April 5, 2003.

CHAPTER 7: THE KENYAN SIDE

1   Stephanie Nolen, "Sex Slaves for Science?" *Globe and Mail*, January 7, 2006.

2   Bwayo's cutting-edge research was in the mid-1990s around HIV and truck drivers. Two articles published on these findings were: J.J. Bwayo, M.A. Omari, A.N. Mutere, W. Jaoko, C. Sekkade-Kigondu, J. Kreiss, and F.A. Plummer, "Long Distance Truck-drivers 1: Prevalence of HIV-1 and Sexually Transmitted Diseases (STDs)," *East African Medical Journal* 68 (1991): 425–9; J.J. Bwayo, A.N. Mutere, M.A. Omari, J.K. Kreiss, W. Jaoko, C. Sekkade-Kigondu, and F.A. Plummer, "Long Distance Truck-drivers 2: Knowledge and Attitudes on Sexually Transmitted Diseases and Sexual Behaviour," *East African Medical Journal* 68 (1991): 714–9.

CHAPTER 9: LEGITIMIZING CIRCUMCISION

1   Two other clinical trials on circumcision were carried out simultaneously to the UNIM trial. One was at Orange Farm in South Africa, conducted by the French National Agency for Research on AIDS. The other was in the Rakai District of Uganda, undertaken by researchers from Johns Hopkins University in Baltimore and Uganda's Makerere University.

2   R.C. Bailey, S. Moses, C.B. Parker, K. Agot, I. Maclean, J.N. Krieger, C.F.M. Williams, R.T. Campbell, and J.O. Ndinya-Achola, "Male Circumcision for HIV Prevention in Young Men in Kisumu, Kenya: A Randomised Controlled Trial," *Lancet* 369, 9562 (2007): 643–56.

3   Epstein, *Invisible Cure*, 266.

4   Speculation about the correlation between circumcision and HIV comes up in a number of articles, including the following: S. Moses, F.A. Plummer, J.E. Bradley, J.O. Ndinya-Achola, N.J.D. Nagelkerke, and A.R. Ronald, "The Association Between Lack of Male

Circumcision and Risk for HIV Infection: A Review of the Epidemiological Data," *Sexually Transmitted Diseases* 21 (1994): 201–10; S. Moses, R.C. Bailey, and A.R. Ronald, "Male Circumcision: Assessment of Health Benefits and Risks," *Sexually Transmitted Infections* 74 (1998): 368–73.

5   John Bongaarts, with Priscilla Reining, Peter Way, and Francis Conant, "The Relationship Between Male Circumcision and HIV Infection in African Populations," *AIDS* 3, 6 (1989): 373–77.

6   S. Moses, J.E. Bradley, N.J.D. Nagelkerke, J.O. Ndinya-Achola, A.R. Ronald, and F.A. Plummer, "Geographical Patterns of Male Circumcision Practices in Africa: Association with HIV Seroprevalence," *International Journal of Epidemiology* 19 (1990): 693–7.

7   Caldwell and Caldwell, "African AIDS Epidemic," 66.

8   Ibid., 68.

9   Gary Slutkin, telephone interviews, July 2010.

10   C.L. Mattson, R.T. Campbell, R.C. Bailey, K. Agot, J.O. Ndinya-Achola, and S. Moses, "Risk Compensation is not Associated with Male Circumcision in Kisumu, Kenya: A Multi-faceted Assessment of Men Enrolled in a Randomized Controlled Trial," *PLoS ONE* 3 (2008): e2443.

CHAPTER 10: UNFINISHED BUSINESS

1   Stella Hryniuk, Report on Annual Review Meeting 2002 of University of Nairobi–University of Manitoba Collaborative Group on STD/AIDS.

2   The program was designed by Stephen Moses, Frank Plummer, and James Blanchard, along with Alix Adrien and Cate Hankins from McGill University in Montreal, and Tota Gangopadhyay from Ottawa.

3 · Other colleagues included Ruth Nduati, James Kiarie, Dalton Wamalwa, Elizabeth Obimbo, Phelgona Otieno, Carey Farquhar, Michael Chung, John Kinuthia, Judd Walson, Walter Jaoko, and Jenn Slyke.

CONCLUSION: AIDS WORLD

1   Donald G. McNeil Jr., "At Front Lines, AIDS War is Falling Apart," *New York Times*, May 10, 2010.

2   Richard Horton, "AIDS: The Elusive Vaccine," *New York Review of Books*, September 23, 2004.

3   Pisani, *Wisdom of Whores*, 124.

4   Ibid., 154.

5   Oldstone, *Viruses, Plagues and History*, 273.

6   Geoffrey York, "A Broken Promise, Paid for in Lives," *Globe and Mail*, June 24, 2010.

7   Peter Piot, interview with the author, London, England, June 2010.

8   John Stover et al., "Can we reverse the HIV/AIDS pandemic with an expanded response?" *Lancet* 360, 9326 (2002): 73–7.

9   S. Moses, F.A. Plummer, E.N. Ngugi, N.J.D. Nagelkerke, A.O. Anzala, and J.O. Ndinya-Achola, "Controlling HIV in Africa: Effectiveness and Cost of an Intervention in a High-frequency STD Transmitter Core Group," *AIDS* 5 (1991): 407–11. In 2010, the Washington-based Results for Development Institute upped the ante with their report, *AIDS2031*, speculating that as much as $733 *billion* would be needed to control AIDS over the next twenty years.

10   Gary Slutkin, telephone interviews with the author, July 2010.

11   Mary Louise Pratt, *Imperial Eyes: Travel Writing and Transculturation* (New York: Routledge, 1992).

12   Ronald et al., "The Nairobi STD Program."

13   Donald G. McNeil Jr., "Advance on AIDS Raises Questions as Well as Joy," *New York Times*, July 26, 2010.

14   Paul McKie, "AIDS Strategy 'Inadequate,'" *Winnipeg Free Press*, April 27, 2002.

Index